Sustainably Improving Health Care

CREATIVELY LINKI
PERFORMANCE, AND

PA
Professor,
Health P
The Geisel Sc
L

T
Associate Profe
Health P
The Geisel Sc
L

American /
a

CULTURE, CONTEXT AND QUALITY IN HEALTH SCIENCES
RESEARCH, EDUCATION, LEADERSHIP AND PATIENT CARE

Series Editors
THOMAS S. INUI AND RICHARD M. FRANKEL

Radcliffe Publishing
London • New York

Radcliffe Publishing Ltd
33–41 Dallington Street
London
EC1V 0BB
United Kingdom

www.radcliffehealth.com

British Library Cataloguing in Publication Data

A catalogue record for this book is available from the British Library.

ISBN-13: 978 184619 521 1

The paper used for the text pages of this book is FSC® certified. FSC (The Forest Stewardship Council®) is an international network to promote responsible management of the world's forests.

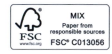

Typeset by Darkriver Design, Auckland, New Zealand
Printed and bound by TJ International Ltd, Padstow, Cornwall, UK

Contents

Contents

Foreword

THERE IS A STICKY MESSAGE AND A SMALL – EVEN BANAL – GRAPHIC image in the construct of this book. It is symbolized by the triangle.

The triangle presents an interesting picture. To some it appears as the capitalized Greek letter delta, a symbol of change; its lowercase version, the small "δ," often represents a differential, as in the difference between desired and current states. Deploying only minimal imagination, one can view the points on the delta or triangle as representing three discrete items – picture the classic three-legged stool. Each of these constructs, products of the simple triangle, is portrayed in this important text edited by Batalden and Foster and enriched by their colleagues.

Clearly, a delta-as-change looms large over the US health-care system and the American public in this decade and the next. However it evolves – as insurance reform, as private enterprise, or government-run system; as an evolution of the important role of all health workers, or as bottom-up, quality-related efforts – it is clear that twenty-first-century medicine will be vastly different than its twentieth-century precedents. What's driving this change? Enumerated elsewhere (and compellingly demonstrated in this book) the changes are the product of many forces: insurance reforms; the quality-improvement-focused accreditation of graduate and continuing education and of health-care systems; an overload – some would say a tsunami – of information, some of which is useful and valid, some not; private and public financial constraints necessitating a hard look at the costs of health care; new understandings about the role of primary care, screening and prevention; and a plethora of reports and calls for quality improvement and patient safety. It is, in fact, a perfect storm of change.

Ironically, the little delta may actually be the most important – if not the biggest – driver of change. Representing the difference between what we should be doing in medicine and what we do, its smallness makes us think of the patient, whose cause we often fail, and whose stories are woven into the fabric of this book. Several additional case examples help paint this picture, using Chassin's descriptions of underuse, overuse, and misuse. An example of overuse, it is apparent that a ubiquitous cancer screening test – the prostate-specific antigen test – is neither an appropriate general screening device nor effectively diagnostic of cancer, leading to unwarranted if well-intended surgery and other treatments, often with unintended outcomes. In contrast, there are many areas of underuse; in cardiovascular disease, for example, many patients recovering from myocardial damage fail to receive proper preventive measures. In mental health, the numbers of patients untreated or undiagnosed for alcoholism, drug addiction, or depression is compelling. Finally there are areas of misuse – the wrong drug for the wrong condition, or several right drugs for right conditions, but each competing with the other – contributing to unwanted outcomes. These are just tiny snapshots of the objects of quality improvement; the text presents many more.

The third manner of viewing the triangle conjures the three-legged stool, each leg represented in the trifold title, *Sustainably Improving Health Care: Creatively Linking Care Outcomes, System Performance, and Professional Development*. The first leg relates to measurement, the root of assessment describing better patient or population outcome. Constructed nationally and applied locally, this leg describes the attempt to measure the burden of illness and its management in quantitative terms. The second leg captures the construct of improvement or better system performance – improving the commitment to and delivery of quality, safety, and value at three levels: the micro, meso, and macro. Finally, the third leg – professional development – is described in a compelling vision of continuing professional formation. The text characterizes this last concept as the root of sustainability, and describes it elegantly, using terms such as mastery, pride, promise, and even joy.

This book makes the persuasive argument that well-intended efforts to redesign and reform health care will enjoy only short lives without the full commitment and engagement of the health-care worker – the product of the sustainability- and capacity-building engine of professional development.

We'll return to the theme of joy shortly.

Triangles and three-legged stools of course occupy space, one in which these three elements have the potential to act synergistically. The book presents practical aspects of this synergism portrayed by descriptions of the Dartmouth-Hitchcock Leadership Preventive Medicine Residency Program, or the development of faculty as coaches – that is, facilitators of the connections in the triangle. This synergistic space is also vividly portrayed in the concept of the Exemplary Practice and Learning Center – an effective practice, teaching, and educational setting described as a potential vehicle for learning in undergraduate medical education. The space is also characterized in terms of governance, leadership, and organization by the experiences of Cincinnati Children's Medical Center, and by an evaluative heuristic in the different cultural setting of Jönköping and southeastern Sweden. Nurses and nurse educators are critical occupiers of the three-point space in this book and in fact in the health-care setting. In the book, much as they do in practice, they offer a candid set of insights as they contemplate the significance of the boundary-spanning invitation of the "triangle" – an invitation filled with both large and small deltas.

There is also a reflective, scholarly, and scientific aspect to this space – the interdisciplinary and necessary science of linking the three in the cause of health-care improvement. This is the interdisciplinary science of health-care improvement; that is, the synergy of integrating the linked aims of outcome measurement, system performance improvement and professional development. Alfred North Whitehead described a profession as work which examines its actions, reflects on them, studies and finds ways to improve them, thus continuously generating new evidence and action. This book lays out for us the beginning of the trans-career, transdisciplinary profession of health-care improvement.

In this context, Whitehead might also ask this question of us: what is the *work* of medicine?

Several years ago, I came across my chief resident in her final year, studying, book-open style, with several patient charts and a clinical practice guideline in front of her. Making notes, getting ready to go home, maybe preparing for an exam, I thought. "What are you doing?" I asked. "Oh," she said, "I'm working on my work." She was reviewing charts to determine how she and other members of our primary care team handled patients, using guideline-driven metrics to assess them, and employing national diabetes standards (if I remember correctly) to learn more. She was, indeed, working on her work.

It is interesting to compare a century-old vision of the work of medicine, exemplified by William Osler, the iconic Canadian/American physician and archetypical medical educator. His life and writings describe the work of the physician embodied in (some would say bounded by) the diagnosis and treatment of disease, the careful history and physical, and the ethical considerations of the doctor-patient relationship – all in a different and much simpler era, to be sure. While brilliant and compelling in Osler's time, Batalden, Foster, and their colleagues urge us to see this view of medicine as the core or substrate of a larger view of the role of the clinician in which we are called to responsibility not only for our own patients but also for our team and the system in which patients and we live and work. It is not that the Oslerian view of work is wrong; it is just that it has been embraced – and in many ways continues to be held firmly – by many current medical educators and the systems which accredit medical education. In contrast to those health professional educators and leaders who appear to believe that if they "get" professional development right, the system will take care of itself, Batalden and Foster leave us with two complementary quotes: "we are responsible for more than just our individual disciplines, intentions, and actions" and "we share responsibilities for outcomes."

However, Osler leaves one lasting image: that of the joyful, happy physician-educator, an image somewhat tarnished today by accounts of the overworked, frustrated clinician. It is a view of medicine for which Batalden and Foster offer the antidote of a more promising, optimistic, even joyful future for the practice of health care.

It is a relatively easy armchair exercise, after reading this book, to imagine other key elements in the future of health care:

- harmonized, continuous certification and licensure
- 360-degree reviews of our activities by patients and team members
- the medical school without walls
- patients, workplace, and evidence as the curriculum for continuing professional development
- meaningful and immediate data collection and feedback
- distributed workplace settings conducive to team collaboration, optimal care, and patient comfort
- meaningful cross-continuum and cross-professional accreditation of educational and health-care systems
- best evidence at the point of care
- seamless, iterative blending of outcomes, improvement, and professional development.

All these and more become part of the new work of medicine!

Last, a conclusion about this text. The clever and sticky message of the triangle reveals itself here not as a banal image but one full of implications for those of us – health-care workers, policy makers, administrators, and patients – who contribute to the culture of academic medical centers and who care about the system. In the journey from twentieth-century Oslerian medicine to some future utopian system or care setting described here, this book, marked by a triangle, will be a milestone.

Dave Davis, MD, CCFP, FCFP
American Association of Medical Colleges
and Toronto University
July 2012

Preface

IDEAS, THEORIES, AND MODELS ARISE FROM MANY SOURCES. MODERN neuroscience suggests that we retain fragments of information, data that we subsequently combine and re-combine. This book is about a model that has emerged from our own work, our observations of the work of colleagues and others, and our reflections about the requirements for the future of the continual improvement of health care. We explore its origins, its content and manifestations, and its implications, particularly for health professional leaders interested in the ongoing improvement of health care. Form and vitality develop in the model as it engages reality – the reality of trying to create cultures of sustainable, generative approaches to the ongoing improvement of health care.

The model links improved care outcomes, improved system performance, and improved professional development. The three linked aims can be graphically represented as a triangle. It is grounded in the lived experience of skilled health professionals and leaders trying to create and deliver good care – while also trying to improve that care.

The authors have different relationships to this idea, but all write from the experience of real work in real settings with real patients and families. All have worked to improve health care and/or have tried to help others understand how to improve health care. They bring diverse perspectives. Chapter 1 provides an overview of the temporal development of the model. Chapters 2, 3, and 4 describe the "corners" of the triangle and their relationships to one another. Chapter 5 explores the way the model has been explicitly embodied in a graduate medical education program. Chapter 6 explores the relation of the linked aims to the simple, complicated, and complex situations faced in the improvement of real care settings. Chapter 7 opens the role of faculty as coaches in the formation of developing practitioners using the model. Chapter 8 offers the chief executive officer's perspective on the challenge of linking the aims into a culture of improvement in an organization. Chapter 9 explores ways of introducing the triangle to undergraduate medical education. Chapter 10 builds on the experiences of changing nursing education to link the aims expressed in the triangle. Chapter 11 uses the model as a heuristic to evaluate and examine a regional improvement in cancer care in southeastern Sweden. Chapter 12, written by the editors, is a reflective inquiry of the chapter authors' own understanding of the triangle as they were writing their chapters. Each lens applied to the idea allows more to be seen.

We have written this book together. We have met regularly and have repeatedly reviewed each other's drafts. When more than a single author is indicated for a chapter, the first author for each chapter has had the lead responsibility for the chapter.

We have benefitted from the facilitative assistance of Ms. Joy McAvoy and the forbearance of our partners and families as we have "had this book and its message deeply on our minds."

We know that all models are wrong and are not the same as the reality they represent. We also know that some models are useful in the daily work of health care and its improvement. We have written this book to invite you to explore these linked aims in your situation. We hope you will test it, build on it, and revise it as you engage the important social task of making health care better.

Paul Batalden
Tina Foster
July 2012

About the Editors

Paul Batalden teaches about the leadership of improvement of health-care quality, safety, and value at The Dartmouth Institute for Health Policy and Clinical Practice, the Institute for Healthcare Improvement (IHI) and The Jönköping Academy for the Improvement of Health and Welfare in Sweden. He chairs the Improvement Science Development Group of The Health Foundation in London. Previously he founded, created, or helped develop the IHI, the US Veterans Administration National Quality Scholars program, the IHI Health Professions Educational Collaborative, the General Competencies of the Accreditation Council for (US) Graduate Medical Education, the Center for Leadership and Improvement in The Dartmouth Institute for Health Policy and Clinical Practice, the Dartmouth-Hitchcock Leadership Preventive Medicine Residency, the Health Professional Faculty Symposium ("summer camp") and the SQUIRE publication guidelines for publishing studies about the improvement of health care. He is a member of the Institute of Medicine of the US National Academy of Sciences. He is currently interested in the multiple knowledge systems that inform the improvement of health and health care.

Tina Foster is Associate Professor of Obstetrics and Gynecology and Community and Family Medicine at The Geisel School of Medicine at Dartmouth. She is a graduate of the University of California San Francisco medical school, and holds a master's degree in public health from the Harvard School of Public Health and master's in science from Dartmouth's Center for Clinical Evaluative Sciences. She is a graduate of the VA National Quality Scholars Fellowship program. She is currently the program director of the Dartmouth-Hitchcock Leadership Preventive Medicine residency program and Associate Director of Graduate Medical Education at Dartmouth-Hitchcock Medical Center. She teaches about health-care improvement and clinical microsystems at The Dartmouth Institute for Health Policy and Clinical Practice. She also serves as Division Director of General Obstetrics and Gynecology at Dartmouth-Hitchcock. Her work is focused on education about the improvement of health care, integrating the Accreditation Council for Graduate Medical Education/American Board of Medical Specialties competencies in undergraduate, graduate, and continuing medical education, and developing knowledge about what it takes to improve the quality, safety, and value of health care.

List of Contributors

James Anderson, JD
Former President and CEO, Cincinnati Children's Hospital Medical Center, Cincinnati, OH, USA

Boel Andersson Gäre, MD, PhD
Director, Futurum, Jönköping County Council and Professor, The Jönköping Academy for Improvement of Health and Welfare, Jönköping, Sweden

Maren Batalden, MD, MPH
Senior Medical Director for Inpatient Quality, Cambridge Health Alliance; Instructor, Harvard Medical School, Boston, MA, USA

Paul Batalden, MD
Professor, The Dartmouth Institute for Health Policy and Clinical Practice, The Geisel School of Medicine at Dartmouth, Hanover, NH, USA; Visiting Professor, The Jönköping Academy for Improvement of Health and Welfare, Jönköping, Sweden

Jeremiah R. Brown, PhD, MS
Assistant Professor, The Dartmouth Institute for Health Policy and Clinical Practice, The Geisel School of Medicine at Dartmouth, Hanover, NH, USA

John Butterly, MD
Associate Professor of Medicine, The Geisel School of Medicine at Dartmouth, Hanover, NH, USA

Thomas A. Colacchio, MD
Immediate Past President, Dartmouth-Hitchcock Medical Center, Lebanon, NH, USA; Professor of Surgery, The Geisel School of Medicine at Dartmouth, Hanover, NH, USA

Linda R. Cronenwett, PhD, RN, FAAN
Beerstecher-Blackwell Professor and Former Dean, University of North Carolina School of Nursing, Chapel Hill, NC, USA

Dave Davis, MD, CCFP, FCFP
Senior Director, Continuing Education and Performance Improvement, Association of American Medical Colleges, Washington, DC, USA; Adjunct Professor, Family and Community Medicine and Health Policy Management and Evaluation, University of Toronto, Toronto, ON, Canada

Tina Foster, MD, MPH, MS
Director, Dartmouth-Hitchcock Leadership Preventive Medicine Residency; Associate Professor, The Geisel School of Medicine at Dartmouth, Hanover, NH, USA

Linda Headrick, MD, MS
Senior Associate Dean for Education, Helen Mae Spiese Distinguished Faculty Scholar and Professor of Medicine, University of Missouri School of Medicine, Columbia, MO, USA

Göran Henriks, MBA
Chief Executive of Learning and Innovation, Qulturum, Jönköping County Council, Jönköping, Sweden

Jonathan Huntington, MD, PhD
Senior Resident, Dartmouth-Hitchcock Leadership Preventive Medicine Residency, Dartmouth-Hitchcock Medical Center, Lebanon, NH, USA

Pamela M. Ironside, PhD, RN, FAAN, ANEF
Professor and Director of the Center for Research in Nursing Education, Indiana University School of Nursing, Indianapolis, IN, USA

Felicia Gabrielsson Järhult, PT, PhD candidate
Physiotherapist, Doctoral Student, The Institute for Gerontology, Jönköping University, Jönköping, Sweden

Kathryn B. Kirkland, MD
Associate Director and Coach, Dartmouth-Hitchcock Leadership Preventive Medicine Residency; Hospital Epidemiologist, Dartmouth-Hitchcock Medical Center, Lebanon, NH, USA; Associate Professor of Medicine, The Geisel School of Medicine at Dartmouth, Hanover, NH, USA

Rosalind A. Lasky, RN, BSN, MS
Health Care Integrator, Section of General Internal Medicine, Dartmouth-Hitchcock Medical Center, Lebanon, NH, USA

List of Contributors

David Leach, MD
Executive Director Emeritus, Accreditation Council for Graduate Medical Education, Chicago, IL, USA

Stephen Liu, MD, MPH
Associate Director, Dartmouth-Hitchcock Leadership Preventive Medicine Residency; Hospitalist, Dartmouth-Hitchcock Medical Center, Lebanon, NH, USA

Charlotte Lundgren, PhD
Associate Professor in Linguistics, Department of Culture and Communication, Linköping University, Sweden

Melanie Mastanduno, BSN, MPH
Director, Population Health Measurement, The Dartmouth Institute for Health Policy and Clinical Practice, Lebanon, NH, USA; Instructor, The Geisel School of Medicine at Dartmouth, Hanover, NH, USA

Craig N. Melin, MBA, MS
President and Chief Executive Officer, Cooley Dickinson Hospital, Northampton, MA, USA

Eugene C. Nelson, DSc, MPH
Co-Director, Center for Population Health, The Dartmouth Institute for Health Policy and Clinical Practice and Professor, The Geisel School of Medicine at Dartmouth, Hanover, NH, USA

Greg Ogrinc, MD, MS
Senior Scholar, White River Junction VA Quality Scholars Program; Associate Professor of Community and Family Medicine and of Medicine, The Geisel School of Medicine at Dartmouth, Hanover, NH, USA

Rune Sjödahl, MD, PhD, FRCS
Professor Emeritus of Surgery, Department of Clinical and Experimental Medicine, The Faculty of Health Sciences, Linköping University, Sweden

Mark E. Splaine, MD, MS
Director, Center for Leadership and Improvement, The Dartmouth Institute for Health Policy and Clinical Practice, Lebanon, NH, USA; Associate Professor of Medicine and Community and Family Medicine, The Geisel School of Medicine at Dartmouth, Hanover, NH, USA

Gautham Suresh, MD, DM, MS
Director, Neonatal Intensive Care Unit, Dartmouth-Hitchcock Medical Center; Coach, Dartmouth-Hitchcock Leadership Preventive Medicine Residency, Lebanon, NH, USA; Associate Professor of Pediatrics, The Geisel School of Medicine at Dartmouth, Hanover, NH, USA

Johan Thor, MD, MPH, PHD
Director, The Jönköping Academy for the Improvement of Health and Welfare, Jönköping, Sweden

The Evolutionary Beginnings of the Model

Paul Batalden

The presenters at a recent improvement conference were describing all the improvement teams in their organization and the challenges of actually improving outcomes for patients. They were getting more and more animated as they described the growing maze of logistics needed to support their efforts. I had just met some well-motivated mid-career physicians and nurses who were trying to improve their care and they were frustrated, finding it hard to get the interest and attention of colleagues that everyone respected. Something clicked as I considered these two "conversations" and I began to listen with different ears, suddenly able to hear and see the fatigue induced by improvement exhortations and endless measurement. I had new insights into the burnout of the good doctors and nurses I met. I heard about the limited successes and frustrations of leaders trying to "incentivize" participation in improvement efforts in a new way. I realized that our invitations to participate in the improvement of care were adding one more thing to already over-full health professionals' lives. We were coming at this from the social and organizational need, bringing real excitement about ever-new ways of doing this work. But we were not engaging professionals in the improvement of health care from within their own efforts to have a meaningful professional life. I realized we needed to rethink what we were doing, if we hoped to create a sustainable, generative process of improvement.

During the twentieth century, new ways of creating better quality, safety, and value were developed in both manufacturing and service sectors of the economy. As the leaders of these changes advocated new ways of measuring and new ways of analyzing and changing work, generalizable notions and theories of work, workplace, worker, and beneficiaries of work emerged.[1-6]

> At the seminar I attended in Atlanta, GA, in 1981, W. Edwards Deming was talking about ball bearings, manufacturing processes, and measurement. I began to wonder why my physician colleague and I had come. The room was full of engineers, some of whom were smoking. We seemed to be the only health professionals. What did all this have to do with health care? That night, my colleague and I took Dr. Deming to dinner. He talked of his experience with his wife's Alzheimer's care and the health professionals and the care settings. The next day, I realized his message was not about ball bearings, manufacturing processes, and measurement: it was about an underlying theory of work, worker, and workplace. Ball bearings and manufacturing were only the language being used.

For these quality pioneers, the phenomenon "quality" included the quality, safety, and value of services and products, and when all of these were at stake, it was clear that it was a matter of design. These key characteristics of the product or service were central to the creation and production of the work itself. Quality was no longer just the concern of inspectors and regulators. Because "quality" connected to every aspect of an organization, it became increasingly clear that it was part of the work of top leadership and the way entire organizations functioned.

As these phenomena became manifest in health care, new approaches to improve and change were connected to new ways of measuring outcomes in individuals and in populations. New roles and processes for accrediting, regulating, and standard-setting bodies emerged.[7–9] Exploring the "usual" ways of work in these new ways revealed nearly infinite opportunities for change and redesign.

> One day my nurse colleague Connie said, "You know you draw the same pictures about the anatomy and about your recommendations for surveillance for the parents of these little girls with their first urinary tract infection and I stand outside at the desk and complete the same lab forms and instructions for collecting urine cultures … What if we printed some of this out ahead and asked the parents to fill in the demographic information on the slips – so we could use our time to have more complete, more effective, and more efficient conversations with them?" She was inviting me to explore and change the process I used in my professional work as a physician.

By the closing decades of the last century, these new ways of making improvement were exploding. Methods for teaching about health care as process and system, about measurement for learning and for reducing unwanted variation, and about facilitating and leading the work of small, multidisciplinary groups working at the front lines of health care became widely available.

Early-adopter leaders realized the possibilities and committed themselves and their organizations to action. Gradually "Flowcharting 101" became process literacy; "Meeting Management 102" became more effective work teams; "Customer Expectations and Satisfaction Measurement 103" became better focus on patient outcomes. Work on the "processes-as-they-were" made people realize the inherent unreliability, undependability, and unwanted variation that was rampant in health care. It was fun to see the discovery and satisfaction that came from being able to make a change and learn from it.

Connecting this newfound local process literacy with generalizable science and the improvement of clinical outcomes began to push our understandings of the complexity of it all.

> In 1984, we started with improving the care for patients who were having hip replacements. The process of selecting the patients, anticipating the rehabilitation and recovery processes, selecting the most appropriate prosthesis, and so forth revealed how interwoven and how many choices were a part of routine patient care. As we moved to other conditions and mapped those processes we began to recognize patterns of changes that could be considered for any clinical process.[10] We also began to recognize the emerging cacophony around outcome measurement, leading us to think of a generalizable frame for these measurements we called a "value compass."[11]

We were realizing that designing and testing changes that attracted local energy and resources was an almost infinitely creative challenge. The love of the challenge attracted wonderful colleagues ... and their excitement and enthusiasm helped their local communities join in the early change-creating work.

Networks of early adopters emerged to facilitate exchanges of learning. Sharing occurred at all levels in health-care service settings: chief executive officers, chief medical officers, chief nursing officers, and those in quality improvement resource jobs – "coaches" and facilitators of the changes. People were proud of what they were learning and were eager to share their insights with others. Consultants were busy at work – with few in health care initially. In a relatively short time, that changed and soon there were consultants of every kind available.

National and international forums were started. Soon there were established connections within and across organizations, local communities, and countries. A common spirit of cooperation and discovery characterized the emerging community of practice. Presentations of the "best local work" were given with pride and received with gratitude ... soon to be adapted and tried elsewhere. By many measures, it was an impressive first decade or so. People really seemed to understand by the systems and processes at work in producing the results caused (in part) health-care outcomes.

These new ways of understanding complex work were almost endless. One top leader team in a hospital got so interested in understanding the process of getting a snack for patients in the middle of the night that they spent 9 months flowcharting all the possibilities! Once we understood how profound our "process illiteracy" was and how much variation there was from day to day and patient to patient, we began to get curious about all the "special cause" contributors and to the myriad "common cause" contributors of that observed variation. The people with the most insight were usually those closest to the work – but they were busy health professionals, many of who were in voluntary organizations. None of this was yet being taught in undergraduate or graduate health professional education. How was this going to remain vital for the long term?

In local settings, the first invitation to health professionals to participate was met with some skepticism, but the allure of "new knowledge" and "new ways of looking at familiar issues and problems" attracted the curiosity and creativity of the health professional community that knew change was needed but had struggled to make it happen. The second invitation to participate in the work of improvement was more focused and sophisticated. The third was recognizable as "one of the interesting ways we do things here." The fourth and fifth began to feel like all-too-familiar exhortations to do more and more. People were beginning to wonder how many invitations they should accept for their lunch hours, their days, and their shifts off. Soon it became possible to discern signs of "improvement fatigue." Slowly it became more difficult to get the right people involved, teams took longer to get their meetings scheduled, intervals between team meetings got so long that it became hard to remember exactly what had happened at the last meeting. In some places, "forming an improvement team/project" became code-talk for slowing things down, or for eventually letting things die of process-correct exploration.

A colleague had just gotten an example of this new way of looking at the work and successfully introducing a change in a high-impact journal! As he debriefed the experience, he described how none of the peer reviewers thought he should mention anything about the process analysis, nor should he mention anything about iterative cycles of change that he had actually used, nor should he use so many time-ordered data sets and analytic statistics to explain the variation he encountered, nor should he talk about the multidisciplinary teams he had assembled to work on the overall process, nor should he describe anything about the context in which these changes were brought about. The "quality" journals wanted examples of "audits" or "medical care evaluation studies" or other "assessment" reports. How was this activity going to develop as a form of science? The usual peer-reviewed scientific health-care literature was not yet very helpful.

Realizing that differences in outcome in differing settings came from differences in systems and processes in differing and particular local contexts challenged our dominant ways of reporting about improvement – as a science. Peer review-ers and editors wanted reports of controlled experiments – but each setting had its own identity and that identity was often in a reflexive interaction with the interventions that were being tested! We were confronting the paradox of seek-ing the development of this new work as science in an epistemological tradition that seemed inimical to that development! Peer-reviewed publications were the language of the professional education community. The high-impact journals were set up to screen out the early reports, but a few health professional educa-tors were beginning to take notice and had begun to explore teaching these ideas despite already over-stuffed curricula. Those teachers began to network and to work as a community of practice.

> The first time that the Dartmouth–Institute for Healthcare Improvement health professional faculty summer symposium ("summer camp") met we realized that it was so easy to insult one another's discipline that we had to practice civil conversation! We quickly realized that we had to attend to much more than respectful communication across health professional disciplines: what united and inspired us was the opportunity to create a commons that allowed us to learn across our disciplines about the redesign of health care. Over the early years, we came to agreement that there were eight knowledge and skill domains that should characterize the learning we were facilitating as teachers of nurses, physicians, and health administrators.[12]

One of those who took notice was David Leach, who became the executive direc-tor of the Accreditation Council for Graduate Medical Education in the United States. This organization sets standards for all specialty education in medicine. He set out to link the processes of professional education with outcomes for those professionals and for their patients: "Good learning for good patient care" became the watchword. Defining the desired outcomes included defining a set of general competencies: Patient Care, Medical Knowledge, Practice-based Learning and Improvement, Professionalism, Interpersonal and Communication Skills, and Systems-based Practice.

It was becoming clearer that the health-care outcomes for individuals and populations, the system quality, safety and value performance, and the develop-ment and formation of health professionals themselves were all linked, given the critical role that professionals themselves actually played in day-to-day care and its reflexive effect on the formation of the professional in development.

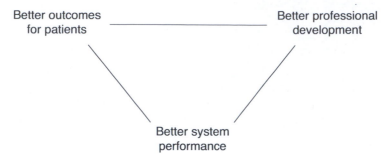

FIGURE 1.1 Linked aims

The inextricable connections among better outcomes, better system performance, and better professional development were becoming visible, and those connections could be instrumental in forming a stable, generative framework for ongoing, creative efforts.

> Parker Palmer had written about the "courage to teach" and had invited attention to the importance of getting the "whole professional – hands, head and heart" to show up for work.[13] He was talking about K-12 teachers, but in reality he was inviting consideration of what made professionals feel "really alive" in their lives and work. He invited attention to the soul of the professional – the inner professional, a deeply personal "solo." But this attention to the "inner professional" in health care was not a soloist phenomenon. The formation of health professionals was importantly influenced by the deeply personal interactions between professional and patient and the contexts in which they came together. The sense of personal and professional mastery that was part of professional competence for health professionals and that offered pride and joy in work involved understanding and designing the situations of health care – as W. Edwards Deming was focusing on as his nearly century-long life and teaching was nearing its end.

Meanwhile, frustrations about the increasingly recognizable gaps between the magnitude of the problems in health care and the ability to execute real change that would close those gaps led to an escalation of the language used to talk about change. "Transformational" change for some meant "change on steroids" or "profound change" or "radically different change." Steps were offered to guide people toward "truly transformative changes." But trying harder didn't seem to make sense – people were really working hard and making their best efforts already! People couldn't imagine where the energy or the resources would come from.

A group of health professionals from Kosovo were visiting Dartmouth and at lunch, one of the visiting surgeons leaned across the table and somewhat sheepishly asked, "Tell me, how can you Americans spend so much money in health care?" I paused for a moment and said, "It's easy, you just need more categories."

We were beginning to think about the synergies of linked aims: better outcomes, better system performance, and better professional development. Bringing them together might offer more energy and less cost/resource use. Taken together these three linked aims could be thought of as a "triangle" capable of creating energy around the ongoing need to improve.

If we thought about these three aims as *inextricably linked* together, was there anyone *not* involved? This was no longer the work of an isolated quality department or a teacher in a survey course. Moving the focus to *everyone* was consistent with the understanding that patients and providers were part of the same systems. This might actually be a model for *transforming* the improvement of health care: different people, different aims for really different results.

How might that be made real? Could we create a model that actually did that? Were there demonstrations that could illustrate how such a model could be made "real"? Alone among the graduate medical specialties, preventive medicine explicitly incorporated formal graduate education and a required practicum to demonstrate the competence in practice. Across the diverse subdivisions of the specialty there was a concern for the health of populations, leadership, systems, and measurement. Over dinner with the leadership of the Accreditation Council for Graduate Medical Education, the elements of a new kind of residency emerged – one that took advantage of the model and the local strengths at Dartmouth-Hitchcock Medical Center and the Dartmouth Institute for Health Policy and Clinical Practice. The seeds of the model-synthesis idea could be sown early in the professional lives of professionals actively forming their own "sense of self." Another opportunity seemed to exist in southern Sweden. (Both of these are described in subsequent chapters of this book.)

Once the model and its linkages were graphically represented, more questions connecting the idea to the real world emerged (*see* Figure 1.2).

Every element and every linkage raised opportunities for inquiry: theory, application, and integration. Each element and linkage invited reflection on the cultures and practices of everyday settings in which professionals and beneficiaries of their work meet. More opportunities for improved performance became immediately visible as the model and the real world met.

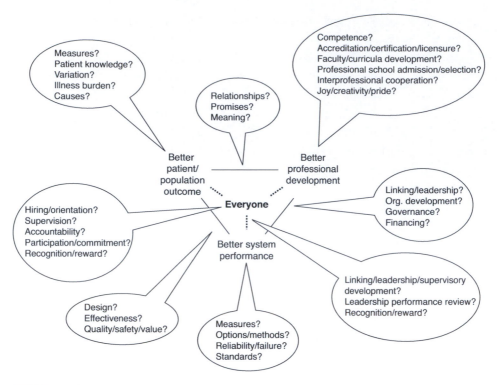

FIGURE 1.2 Questions the model invites

The more we reflected on the model, the more we began to realize that it could be used to contextualize the everyday work of bringing generalizable science into everyday practice. The simple logic reflected in the formula shown in Figure 1.3 is used every day as health professionals seek to translate and apply science to the needs of the people they meet and try to serve.

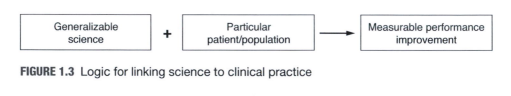

FIGURE 1.3 Logic for linking science to clinical practice

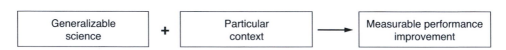

FIGURE 1.4 Logic for linking science to improvement

Substituting the word, "context," for the word, "patient" (*see* Figure 1.4) in this familiar logic offered insight into the challenges of bringing science into practice.[14] We soon realized that each of the elements – word and symbol – in this simple formula denotes a different knowledge system.[15,16] Each knowledge system is constructed differently. Each knowledge system tests the validity and goodness of knowledge built differently. However, "good" improvement requires the integration and use of all the elements. This work of good improvement lives in the context of the systems of professional work and practice.

Framing the work of improvement in the context of the linked aims invites consideration of what might be necessary to sustain truly generative efforts (*see* Figure 1.5).

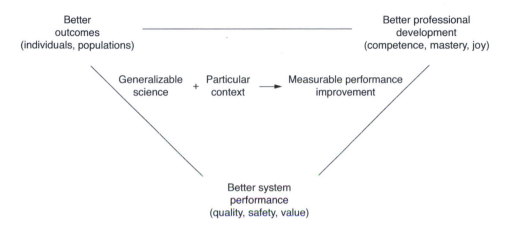

FIGURE 1.5 Connecting improvement work to linked aims

This model invites the recognition of the method and knowledge, skills needed to bring science into daily work and in the service of a set of linked aims, which together contribute to the sustainability of the work of improvement – and to its continuing generativity. The chapters that follow in this book will begin to illustrate this as they open the deeper exploration of these aims and their interdependence.

References

1. Deming WE. *Out of the Crisis.* Cambridge: Massachusetts Institute of Technology Center for Advanced Engineering Study; 1986.
2. Juran JM, Godfrey AB. *Juran's Quality Handbook.* 5th ed. New York, NY: McGraw-Hill; 1999.
3. Crosby PB. *Quality is Free.* New York, NY: McGraw-Hill; 1979.
4. Feigenbaum A. *Total Quality Control.* 3rd ed (revised). New York, NY: McGraw-Hill; 1991.
5. Ishikawa K. *Introduction to Quality Control.* 3rd ed. Tokyo: JUSE Press; 1990.
6. Ishikawa K. *What is Total Quality Control?* Lu DJ, translator. Englewood Cliffs, NJ: Prentice-Hall; 1985.

7. Joint Commission on Accreditation of Healthcare Organizations (JCAHO). *The Measurement Mandate*. Oakbrook Terrace, IL: JCAHO; 1993.
8. Joint Commission on Accreditation of Healthcare Organizations (JCAHO). *Framework for Improving Performance*. Oakbrook Terrace, IL: JCAHO; 1994.
9. Joint Commission on Accreditation of Healthcare Organizations (JCAHO). *Striving Toward Improvement*. Oakbrook Terrace, IL: JCAHO; 1992.
10. Batalden P. The changing times: moving ahead to improving clinical conditions. *Proceedings Hospital Quality Technology Network*; 1993 June 3–4; Aberdeen Woods Conference Center, Peachtree City, GA. Nashville, TN: Hospital Corporation of America; 1993.
11. Nelson EC, Batalden P, *et al*. Improving health care, part 1: the clinical value compass. *Jt Comm J Qual Improv*. 1996; **22**(4): 243–58.
12. Batalden P, Splaine M. What will it take to lead the continual improvement and innovation of health care in the twenty-first century? *Qual Manag Health Care*. 2002; **11**(1): 45–54.
13. Palmer P. *The Courage to Teach*. San Francisco, CA: Jossey-Bass; 2007.
14. Batalden P, Davidoff F. What is "quality improvement" and how can it transform health care? *Qual Saf Health Care*. 2007; **16**(1): 2–3.
15. Batalden P, Bate P, Webb D, *et al*. Planning and leading multidisciplinary colloquium to explore the epistemology of improvement. *BMJ Qual Saf*. 2011; **20**(Suppl. 1): i1–4.
16. Batalden P, Davidoff F, Marshall M, *et al*. So what? Now what? Exploring, understanding and using the epistemologies that inform the improvement of healthcare. *BMJ Qual Saf*. 2011; **20**(Suppl. 1): i99–105.

2

Better Patient and Population Outcome

Practical Approaches that Health Systems Can Adopt for Measuring the Health of Patients and Populations

Eugene C. Nelson, John Butterly, Thomas A. Colacchio, Melanie Mastanduno, Tina Foster, and Paul Batalden

Introduction

Sustainable and continuous improvement of health care in both the domains of quality and cost calls for a tripartite focus: better outcomes of care, better system performance, and better professional formation and development. If better health outcomes are to be realized for people, patients, and populations, then it will be necessary to *measure* changes in health status that occur over time. The primary focus of this chapter is on using measures of health to track improvement in health outcomes for individuals and populations served by academic medical centers. We begin the chapter with a case study to frame the issues and to illustrate key principles. Next we explore the topic of measuring health outcomes by discussing a model of health, methods for measuring health, and specific practical measures of health. We conclude the chapter with a brief discussion on integrating the "outcomes" point of the triangle with the other two points and with a warning about problems that could arise if we were to place too much emphasis on measuring health outcomes and miss the point of improving or optimizing the actual health experienced by people, patients, and populations.

Section 1: Dartmouth-Hitchcock Case Example
• •

The product of a health system should be health.

—Thomas Colacchio, MD,
President Emeritus, Dartmouth-Hitchcock

This case describes the work of Dartmouth-Hitchcock (DH) to improve patient outcomes and population health. DH is an integrated health system including a rural academic medical center that employs over 900 physicians and 7000 staff and which serves approximately 1.2 million people living in New Hampshire and eastern Vermont.

Vision, Strategy, and Tactics

The vision of DH is to "achieve the healthiest population possible, leading the transformation of health-care in our region and setting the standard for the nation."[1] The strategy is to deliver the highest value health care to the populations that DH serves. Key tactics are to (a) measure the value of health care, defined as the health outcomes and care experiences of patients and populations in relationship to health costs incurred over time, and (b) build the capability of all clinicians, administrators, and employees to use improvement science to continuously increase the value of their work.

Strategic Execution: Circles of Influence on Patient and Population Health

The DH strategic plan for population health is based on the concept of circles of influence and is illustrated in Figure 2.1. The center of the target represents the vision-strategy-tactic trio described earlier. Moving out from the center, there are a series of concentric circles that depict populations on which DH has influence; as we move from the inner to the outer rings, the potential for influence diminishes. The logic underlying the circles of influence is that the health system has the potential for the most direct and substantial impact on the health of and value creation for its own employees and their families, as well as significant impact on its primary care and specialty care patients. The impact may be somewhat less for the accountable care organization (ACO) populations that use the DH health system as a major (but not necessarily sole) source of health-care. Meanwhile, by partnering with communities and other stakeholders (such as public health officials, employers, payers, educators, researchers, politicians, policy makers, communication specialists) both regionally and nationally, DH can influence the factors that contribute to the health status and the value of care for non-DH-served populations residing in the region and the rest of the country.

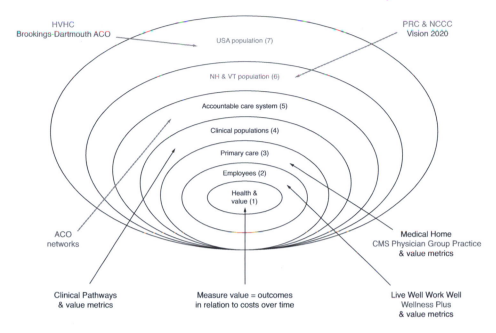

FIGURE 2.1 Specific population health programs to advance the Dartmouth-Hitchcock Medical Center strategy

First Steps: Using New Programs and Standard Measures to Improve Patient and Population Health

To move from good intentions to effective execution, DH is taking steps to start new programs that will advance patient and population health and embed standard measures of health and value into the operations of the programs and the flow of health care. These steps are shown in Table 2.1.

TABLE 2.1 Summary of Dartmouth-Hitchcock Medical Center (DHMC) Strategic Programs and Measures of Health and Value

Population	Program Name	Population Estimate	Health and Value Measures*			
			Risk	Disease	Function	Costs
DHMC employees, families, and retirees	Live Well/Work Well DH Wellness Plan	15 000	X	X	X	X
DHMC primary care	Patient-centered medical homes	100 000		X	X	X
DHMC specialty care	High Value Healthcare Programs and Pathways	300 000		X	X	X

(continued)

Population	Program Name	Population Estimate	Health and Value Measures*			
			Risk	Disease	Function	Costs
DHMC ACO	DH ACO	100 000		X	X	X
NH and VT residents	Prevention Research Center at Dartmouth	1 500 000	X	X	X	X
US residents	High Value Healthcare Collaborative	300 000 000	X	X	X	X
	Dartmouth Atlas Project					
	Advanced ACO network					

Notes: *The "X" in the last four columns denotes measures that are being collected or that are planned for collection. ACO, accountable care organization; DH, Dartmouth-Hitchcock; NH, New Hampshire; VT, Vermont.

Employees, Families, and Retirees

Two new and related programs serve the groups of employees, families, and retirees. One of these is Live Well/Work Well, a program that aims to improve the health and productivity of employees and their families while decreasing their health-care costs. It offers an annual health assessment, health coaching, and a wide variety of occupational health and health promotion services. Another is the Dartmouth-Hitchcock Wellness Plus employer-based program, which offers complementary services including care management and population management services (such as identifying people in need of chronic care or preventive services) in addition to personalized assistance navigating the insurance plan. Standard measures that are designed into these programs reflect health outcomes (risk, functional, and disease status) and per capita health-care costs.

Primary Care Patients

DH is transforming its collection of conventional primary care practices, based in 25 different locations, into patient-centered health homes with common care models, core processes, clinical pathways, and care management services. These require standard measures of health outcomes, patient experience, and per capita health-care costs to enable the creation of common balanced scorecards. These sites (all of which have achieved National Committee for Quality Assurance[2] level III status) have been effectively transformed into functioning medical homes, facilitated by DH's participation as one of 10 health-care organizations in the Centers for Medicare and Medicaid Services (CMS) Physician Group Practice Demonstration Project. They have a leadership council consisting of primary care leaders, system leaders, and patients and family members that provides planning and oversight to strategic improvements and operations. A primary care "collaboratory" engages all the practice sites and uses standard measures to determine which practices have the best results, facilitating understanding and dissemination of standard processes that produce best measured outcomes.[3]

"Homegrown" internal improvement experts (quality improvement professionals) who are embedded in each practice and who receive ongoing education to increase their improvement coaching expertise facilitate the work of the primary care collaboratory.

Specialty Care Patients

DH is rapidly developing programs for major clinical populations, such as spine conditions, total joint replacement, diabetes, heart failure, perinatal care, depression, breast cancer, and end-of-life care. This action-learning approach engages frontline staff and patients to redesign care for best value. It works by (a) standardizing core processes based on the best available evidence, (b) engaging patients in shared decision making and self-management, and (c) using health information technology for decision support, for clinical population management, and to contribute "data points" to quality, outcomes, and cost measurement. Feedforward and feedback patient-reported measures are an important facet of these care programs,[4] as well as formal action-learning programs to coach value improvement in mesosystems of care (the set of clinical microsystems that provide care to clinical populations across the continuum and over time) and to track health outcomes and costs.[5]

Dartmouth-Hitchcock Accountable Care Organization Patients

DH is developing ACO programs by working with multiple payers to move away from fee-for-service payments and toward value-based payments.[6] Having some payers reward DH for better value while others pay for higher volumes is not in the best interests of the communities served by DH nor does it reflect the professional values of DH. Following its initial successes in the value-based Medicare demonstration program (the CMS-Physician Group Practice Demonstration Project) and now embarking on a new CMS pioneer ACO program, additional contracts have been negotiated with commercial payers (CIGNA, Anthem, Harvard Pilgrim Health Care) that align with the new CMS guidelines for ACO payments. In general, these contracts reward better quality and lower per capita costs based on comparative measures of performance.

New Hampshire and Vermont Residents

Because health is determined by many factors in addition to health care (social environment, physical environment, behavioral patterns),[7] DH and related organizations (The Dartmouth Institute for Health Policy and Clinical Practice [TDI] and Dartmouth College) are partnering with community groups, employers, public health officials, and others in joint programs to promote health, prevent disease, and minimize the burden of illness in support of the DH vision of the healthiest population possible. Examples of community partnerships for health include the Prevention Research Center at Dartmouth, which aims to improve cardiovascular health in New Hampshire and Vermont, the Norris Cotton Cancer Center community-based prevention program, and the Vision 2020 community health campaign that is underway in Keene, New Hampshire. DH is embedding common measures of health risk and of functional health status into these programs whenever possible.

US Residents

DH is working with TDI to implement two national programs that share the common aim of improving health and value. The High Value Healthcare Collaborative, based on the Dartmouth Spine Center's work to measure and improve value,[8] was started in 2011 with the aim of rapidly improving the value of health care while accelerating the adoption of patient-centered measures of health and efficiency to improve care delivery and accountability. The High Value Healthcare Collaborative is coordinated by TDI and was founded by progressive health systems – Cleveland Clinic, Dartmouth-Hitchcock, Denver Health, Intermountain Health Care, and the Mayo Clinic – and has expanded to include many other health systems. The focus is on use of standard measures of outcomes and costs across all organizations to compare, evaluate, and improve value for major clinical populations (total knee replacement, diabetes, depression, perinatal care, asthma, heart failure, end-of-life care) by observing what processes are generating the best outcomes at lowest costs. The Brookings-Dartmouth ACO program started in 2010 is providing national leadership in forming learning networks to assist ACOs, in establishing measures of performance to be used for value-based payment, and in researching the emergence of ACOs to determine and share knowledge about the factors that contribute to the successful start-up of new ACOs.

Summary

DH and TDI, DH's education, research and demonstration program partner, are promoting a "family" of population health programs that target different populations within the organizations' circles of influence. All of these programs share the aim of improving health and value and all are enhanced by the use of standard, and when possible, equivalent measures of health outcomes and health costs. But what are these standard measures, and what are the associated challenges in developing and using them? In the next part of this chapter, we will address both underlying concepts and specific measures that will be used by DH and others as they face the challenge of understanding the "outcomes" point of the triangle.

Section 2: Measuring Health Outcomes in Patients and Populations

We will now explore critical models, methods, and measures[9] that are hidden beneath the surface of the DH case study presented earlier. We believe that these models, methods and measures are the fundamentals that must be understood and mastered to bring the "outcomes" corner of the triangle fully into play.

A Model of Health and Health Outcomes

Figure 2.2 shows a model of health determinants and outcomes that is based on the work of Evans and Stoddart,[10] the World Health Organization,[11] and others. The model suggests that the health of individuals and populations has multiple determinants including genetic endowment, physical environment, socioeconomic environment, patterns of living and behaving, and health care. These determinants interact with one another and evolve over the course of a lifetime to produce an individual's health status. The health status of an individual has three major domains: (1) risk status, (2) functional status, and (3) disease status. Each of these three health status domains may change as individuals grow older or become ill or injured, as they change their habits and lifestyle, as they receive health care, and as their physical and socioeconomic environment changes around them.

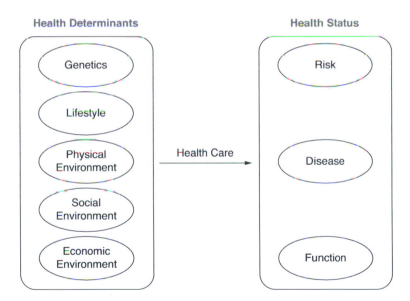

FIGURE 2.2 Determinants of health and health outcomes (source: Madans Jennifer H. The Budapest Initiative: Measuring Population Health Status in Surveys and Censuses. The Joint UNECE/WHO/Eurostat Task Force on Measurement of Health Status. *Presented at the Eurostat Meeting on Disability Statistics.* Dublin, Ireland, September 18, 2007.)

Two features of this model merit further discussion. First, changes in health status from one time in a person's life to a later time in that same person's life are often called "health outcomes." However, strictly speaking, there is really only one *final* health outcome (death); most things that we call "health outcomes" are more accurately seen as changes in health *status* that can be described as changes in risk, functioning, or disease. Second, in general, everyone has a personal (endogenous) health risk status (based on genetics, demographics, biometrics, and behaviors) as well as a personal functional health status (which includes physical function, mental health, and social/role function). However, not everyone has a disease status. For example, anyone who is fortunate enough to be free from acute or chronic disease or permanent disability will have risk and functional statuses but no disease status. This has important implications when we turn our attention to measuring health, because while we can use generic measures of risk and function that apply to everyone, we also need condition-specific measures of disease that apply only to people with a certain, select health problem or constellation of health conditions. The activities described in the DH case use the model of health determinants and health outcomes shown in Figure 2.2 as fundamental planks in the platform of programs that aim to optimize patient and population health and increase value.

Methods for Measuring Health Outcomes

Having introduced a model that brings together determinants of health and domains of health outcomes, we now focus on methods that can be used to collect data on health outcomes and related measures of system performance. The aim of all modern health systems is to produce the best health outcomes (risk status, disease status, functional status) for patients and populations while delivering services that are of the highest possible quality (safe, timely, equitable, effective, efficient, and patient centered) at the lowest total costs to consumers and payers.[12] In short, the aim is to improve the value of the product produced by health systems, where value is defined as health outcomes (reflecting various domains of health status) and health-care quality in relationship to total health-care costs over time.[13]

What prompts interaction with the health system? People live with families and friends in their communities and from time to time they are ill or injured or have a health-care need. At that point they may become patients who enter the health-care system and embark on a health-care *journey*. Figure 2.3 illustrates the idea that people move in and out of the health-care system on short or long journeys that may include stops in many locations such as a primary care medical home or a specialist's office, an emergency department, a community hospital, a nursing home, or a quaternary academic medical center. A mother might take a quick trip with her toddler to see the pediatrician for a sore throat and fever that goes away in a few days or might accompany her teenager on a jaunt to the emergency department for a lacerated elbow that requires a few stitches and which heals rapidly. On the other hand, the journey may be an extended, complex, and arduous safari. Imagine a person with chest pain who goes to the local emergency department and is diagnosed with acute myocardial infarction. He is stabilized and then transported to the academic medical center where he receives a stent in the cardiac catheterization lab. After being transferred to the cardiac care unit and then a few days later to a step-down unit, he is transferred to a nursing home for a 30-day stay and finally enters an outpatient cardiac rehabilitation program that runs for several months.

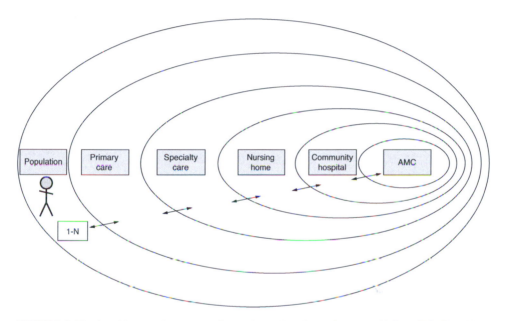

FIGURE 2.3 The health-care journeys of people and patients (source: Nelson EC, Batalden PB, Mohr JJ, *et al*. Building a quality future, *Front Health Serv Manage*, 1998; **15**(1): 3–32. Used with permission of the authors.)

One of the many challenges presented by both long and short journeys is collecting the data along the way, both to provide the best care in the right place at the right time in real time. This challenge is heightened when we consider the simultaneous need to track and to assemble this data over time in order to measure and improve the outcomes and costs of care based on program evaluation, improvement projects, and research programs.

To determine the extent to which the aim of value creation is realized, as well as to improve care, we need to measure health outcomes and the costs of health care for both individual patients and populations at the point of service in real time as care is provided, and to repeat these measures over time to determine the long-term impact of the health-care services delivered on outcomes and costs of care. This requires the design of rich information environments that can feed data forward, to the point of service as care is delivered, and can feed data back to different stakeholders for evaluation, improvement, accountability, and research (*see* Sidebar).[14,15]

The challenge is to make these vital performance measures available both at the point of service and over time for individual patients as well as populations. To achieve this, we must design and implement health information systems that feed forward and feed back core data on changes in health status as well as key indicators of quality and costs. These core data must be drawn from several different sources or data streams, including diagnostic tests from laboratory systems, administrative data from billing and claims systems, clinician reports from health record systems, patient reports from personal health record systems, or patient health assessment portals linked to electronic health records and patient health status surveys. Figure 2.4 provides a diagram that illustrates the use of feedforward and feedback data in the flow of care.

It is essential to recognize that the preferred source for some of the core data is the patient, who is, after all, the primary user and beneficiary of health care. To make a health-care outcomes and value measurement system affordable and practical, there is a need to design health information systems that (1) capture patient-reported data and feed this and other key information (such as diagnoses, diagnostic test results, patient prefer-

Example of a Feedforward and Feedback Data System
A simple example of a feedforward and feedback data system is to make sure that a primary care patient with hypertension always has her prior blood pressure values (as well as her current reading) available when she sees the clinician who is actively treating her hypertension. Feeding the data forward enables the patient and clinician to see how the care plan has affected the level of blood pressure up to this point in time. Then aggregating the data for this particular hypertension patient, as well as for all similar patients treated by the practice for hypertension, can provide data on the degree of success that the provider, or practice, is achieving in helping patients control their blood pressure. Data feedback of this type facilitates assessment of current practice performance and lays the groundwork for measurably determining improvement in performance in the future. This same principle can be extended to capture various data pertinent to health outcomes (e.g., risk status, functional status, disease-specific status) and other data (e.g., decision quality, patient engagement, and health-care costs) and to use the data to create a closed-loop feedforward and feedback information system.

ences and treatments prescribed) forward, as care is delivered; (2) feed back the data to clinicians, patients, families, payers, and regulators to reflect changes in health status associated with health care; and (3) provide performance data on the outcomes and costs of care and services provided to patients and populations. Meeting this challenge could be regarded as an impossible task, but fortunately there are already working examples of health information systems that make use of patient-reported data to make care more effective, more efficient, more

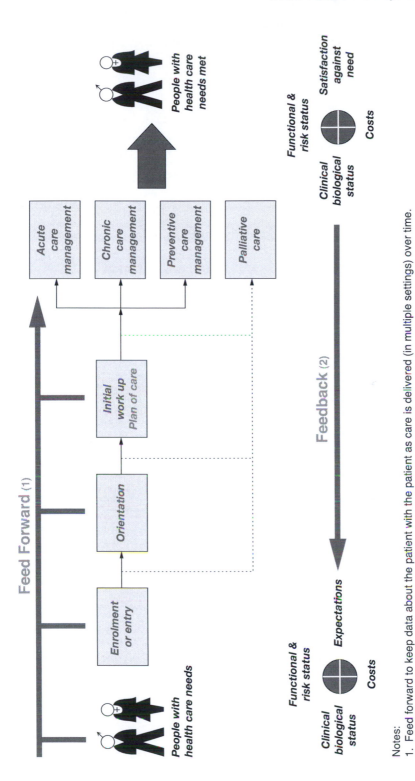

People with
health care needs met

People with
health care needs

Feed Forward (1)

Feedback (2)

Enrolment
or entry

Orientation

Initial
work up
Plan of care

Acute
care
management

Chronic
care
management

Preventive
care
management

Palliative
care

*Functional &
risk status*

Expectations

*Clinical
biological
status*

Costs

*Functional &
risk status*

*Satisfaction
against
need*

*Clinical
biological
status*

Costs

Notes:
1. Feed forward to keep data about the patient with the patient as care is delivered (in multiple settings) over time.
2. Feed back to provide summary data on clinical populations to improve care in individual programs, collaborative networks, and to provide research data base.

FIGURE 2.4 Using feedforward and feedback data in flow of care for patient care, improvement, and research

(© 2000 Trustees of Dartmouth College; used with permission.)

patient centered and more likely to produce the outcomes desired by patients and families.[16]

Specific Practical Measures of Health Outcomes and End-User Value

In the preceding section we discussed the notion of journeys through the health-care system and the need for data collection methods that can generate rich information environments to optimize care as it is delivered by feeding data forward and to improve care for future patients by feeding data back to the system. We now turn to practical measures that can be used to measure health outcomes and health-care value. Table 2.2 provides a summary of the measures and measurement methods that are discussed next.

TABLE 2.2 Practical Methods for Measuring Health Outcomes and Costs

	Domains or Topics	Measurement Methods	Comments
Risk Status	Cardiovascular risk	Framingham Cardiovascular Index	Predicts adults' 10-year risk of death from cardiovascular causes based on demographics and biometrics
	Overall health risk	IHME-Dartmouth Health Risk Index	Predicts adults' 10-year all-cause mortality risk based on demographics, biometrics and health behaviors
Disease Status*	Diabetes	HgbA1c	Blood test that measures the patient's blood sugar level over the past 2–3 months
	COPD	FEV-1	Lung function test that measures the volume of air that the individual can push out of his/her lungs in 1 second
	Depression	PHQ-9	Nine-item self-report scale that measures the severity of depression in adults
	Low back pain	Oswestry Back Pain Disability Index	Sixty-item self-report scale that measures the severity of low back pain
Functional Status#	Physical health, mental health, social role function, overall health	VR-12, VR-36	Twelve- and thirty-six-item self-report scale that measures physical health, mental health, and social role function
	Physical health, mental health, social role function, overall health, quality of life	PROMIS-10, PROMIS-29^	Ten- and twenty-nine-item self-report scale that measures physical health, mental health and social role function
	Physical health, mental health, overall health	EQ-5D and EQ-VAS§	Six-item self-report scale that measures mobility, self-care, usual activities, pain/discomfort, anxiety/depression, and overall health

	Domains or Topics	Measurement Methods	Comments
	Physical health, mental health, social role function, overall health	CDC Healthy Days	Four-item self-report that measures overall health and number of days in past 30 days not in good health or could not do usual activities
Health Costs: Direct	Health-care cost per capita, health-care resource use per capita	Dartmouth Atlas: 65 and older	Medicare health insurance claims based per capita annual measure on actual expenses paid for health-care services and for resources used based on standard prices
	Health-care cost per capita, health-care resource use per capita	Health Partners of Minnesota: under 65	All payer insurance claims based per capita annual measure on actual expenses paid for health-care services and for resources used based on standard prices
Health Costs: Indirect	Health-related work limitations, productivity, presenteeism	WLQ: Work Limitations Questionnaire§	Eight-item self-report scale that measures the degree to which employed individuals are experiencing limitations on the job due to their health problems, and health-related productivity loss
	Health-related work limitations, productivity, presenteeism	WPAI: Work Productivity and Activity Impairment Questionnaire§	Six-item self-report scale that estimates the percentage of time missed due to a health problem, the percentage of impairment while working due to a health problem and the overall percentage of work impairment

Notes: *Illustrative condition-specific measures shown in table; #illustrative measures of functional health status (physical health, mental health, social/role function) shown in table. ^PROMIS measures are open access instruments that were developed with National Institutes of Health funding. PROMIS has both static and dynamic forms. Dynamic form measures for physical health, mental health, and some symptoms (fatigue, sleep, breathing) are available in an open-source, computerized adaptive testing mode that dynamically selects items to ask the respondent based on prior answers and maximizes precision of measurement while minimizing respondent burden. §This measure is copyrighted and licensed; users may be charged licensing fees depending on the owner's policies and use of the instrument. CDC, Centers for Disease Control and Prevention; COPD, chronic obstructive pulmonary disease; EQ-VAS, EQ visual analogue scale; FEV-1, forced expiratory volume in 1 second; IHME, Institute for Health Metrics and Evaluation; PHQ-9, Patient Health Questionnaire depression scale; PROMIS, Patient Reported Outcomes Measurement Information System; VR-12, Veterans RAND 12-Item Health Survey; VR-36, Veterans RAND 36-Item Health Survey.

Measuring Health Risk Status

As noted earlier in this chapter, the health risk of an individual patient or a population has multiple determinants. Some major sources of risk *surround* the individual and are part of his or her physical, social, and economic environment. Other major sources of risk are *within* the individual and are part of his or her personal makeup; these endogenous risk factors include (a) genetic endowment; (b) demographic characteristics such as age, sex, race, and ethnicity; (c) biometric characteristics such as body mass, blood pressure level, blood sugar, cholesterol; and (d) recurrent patterns of behavior or lifestyle such as diet, exercise habits, smoking, alcohol use, and seatbelt use.

While summary measures of health risk have existed for decades, there are relatively few that are valid, reliable, practical, and freely available for use by patients, clinicians, consumers, employers, and others. Two health indices that are fit for practical use and widespread adoption are the Framingham Cardiovascular Index[17] and the Institute for Health Metrics and Evaluation (IHME)-Dartmouth Health Risk Index.[18] The Framingham index is based on epidemiologic data from a large prospective study of factors associated with cardiovascular disease and related deaths. It has been used and refined for decades and has been validated for many different populations. It provides an estimate of the 10-year risk of death from cardiovascular events based on demographic and biometric characteristics.

The IHME-Dartmouth index is based on recent meta-analyses of health risk factors that have been done in the United States and abroad. It has been validated using National Health and Nutrition Examination Survey follow-up study data, a national prospective study of health risks and mortality. The IHME-Dartmouth risk measure is now ready for use in clinical settings and employer- and community-based health and wellness programs. It provides an estimate of the 10-year risk of avoidable death from the leading causes of mortality, and is based on demographic factors, biometric characteristics, and behaviors that confer or reduce risk. It should be noted that the IHME-Dartmouth index is a *generic* measure of health risk and can be applied to all adults between the ages of 30 and 79 whether or not they have a chronic disease or special health problem.

Measuring Disease Status

Disease generally refers to a derangement in the physiological or psychological status of an individual that is associated with pathophysiology.[19] Disease states may be acute or chronic. Transient diseases are sometimes referred to as acute, time-limited problems; examples include a tension headache, the common cold, or a stress reaction brought on by an event but which dissipates quickly. Other diseases have an onset, potential for progression, and do not resolve; rather they become a permanent part of the individual's physiological or psychological makeup and may become progressively worse over time. Permanent diseases are often referred to as chronic problems; examples include congestive heart failure, chronic obstructive pulmonary disease, and Alzheimer's disease. The course of chronic disease progression may be swift, slow, or irregular over time.

There are many valid and practical measures of disease status. For the most part, measures of disease status are specific to a particular disease such as diabetes, asthma, migraine headache, chronic back pain, anxiety, or depression.

Table 2.2 lists a few illustrative common diseases and valid, practical measures that enjoy widespread use. Some of these disease-specific measures use diagnostic test values (e.g., HgbA1c for diabetes). There are also some generic disease metrics, which aim to reflect the overall burden of illness and may be used for case mix adjustment or for predicting future health-care utilization. These are generally based on combining the presence of multiple diseases and disease severity. One such generic, public domain measure is the widely used Charlson Index, based on a count of the number of comorbidities.[20]

Measuring Functional Health Status

Functional health status refers to a person's ability to carry out activities that are part of his or her everyday life. Functional health status may be measured in multiple domains such as physical, mental, and social role functioning, and may be categorized along a continuum of performance in each domain. In general the burden of illness in an individual will be reflected in limitations in functional health; the greater the burden of illness the greater the degree of functional limitations. Therefore, one reason to minimize the burden of illness is to maintain the person's ability to actively and fully engage in their everyday life activities – such as being productive at work or school and taking part in family, social, community, and leisure activities that contribute to the overall perception of wellness.

Over the past decades, scores of functional health status measures have been developed. Some are disease or condition-specific while others are generic and apply to virtually any child or adult. Two of the best and most practical generic measures of functional health status are the VR-12 and VR-36 (Veterans RAND 12- and 13-item health surveys; public domain versions of the SF-12 and SF-36) and the Patient Reported Outcomes Measures and Information System (PROMIS) measures. The VR-12 and VR-36 are well established measures of functional health and can be scored to generate summary indexes of physical health and mental health.[21] The PROMIS measures are newer measures of patient-reported outcomes that have been developed by teams of measurement experts with funding from the National Institutes of Health.[22] PROMIS covers a large number of domains of health within the general rubric of physical, mental and social function. PROMIS measures are available as "static" forms as well as "dynamic" computer-based surveys, which use computerized adaptive testing software to select the shortest list of items to ask to produce a precise measurement of an individual's status on any particular dimension of functional status.

Measuring Costs of Health Care and Health Limitations to Consumers, Payers, and Employers

The costs associated with health conditions can be divided into two major categories. The first category is *direct health-care costs*, which includes payments that are made by the patient or on behalf of the patient to receive health-care services. Direct costs encompass a wide variety of services such as physician care, emergency visits, hospital services, nursing home care, home health care, diagnostic tests, medications, procedures, and medical equipment. The second category is *indirect social costs*, which reflect expenses that are borne by the family, the community, and employers. This includes a wide variety of health-related costs such as informal caregiver costs when services are provided by families and friends and productivity costs due to the inability of a person to go to work for health reasons (absenteeism) or reductions in an employee's ability to do his work even though he is at work (presenteeism).

Methods for measuring direct health-care costs are generally based on the analysis of health-care claims data, such as Medicare claims data or all-payer claims databases that are available in some states and can be used to estimate per capita costs.[23] Though difficult to collect, out-of-pocket costs for health care can be measured based on consumer self-report, as is done in the National Medical Care Expenditure Survey.[24] Methods for measuring the indirect costs of health conditions (real costs borne by society but not reflected in claims data) generally rely on employer records (including days lost from work due to illness/injury, workman's compensations records and long-term disability records) and on employee self-reports on work limitations associated with health conditions. Two widely used self-report measures of productivity are the Work Productivity and Activity Impairment Questionnaire, which measures time missed due to a health problem and the degree of impairment while working due to a health problem, and the Work Limitations Questionnaire, which measures the degree to which employees have job limitations due to health problems and health-related productivity loss.[25,26]

Summary

Although a large variety of validated metrics exist (as described earlier) there are also many challenges to collect them reliably, meaningfully, and efficiently and to use them for both individual patient and clinical population needs. However, it is exceedingly likely that in the near future, high-performing health systems will include health outcomes tracking (using both feedforward and feedback methods) to improve their ability to develop treatment plans best matched to health needs and preferences and to monitor and improve outcomes for individual patients and populations by applying improvement science and comparative effectiveness research as well as other methods.

Section 3: Integrating the Outcomes Point of the Triangle with the Other Two Points
••••••••••••••••••••••••••••••

In this final section we aim to connect the points of the triangle by briefly discussing how improving outcomes relates to improving system performance and professional development.

Improving Outcomes and System Performance

Several critical considerations reflect the linkage between improving outcomes and improving system performance. First, the system of health-care delivery (along with other determinants of health) produces the health outcomes that people desire as well as outcomes that they dread. In brief, good systems produce good outcomes. If we are serious about improving desired health outcomes, we will need to go upstream and understand the system of causes, determine what parts of the system can be changed, make intelligent efforts to design and test these changes, and observe the impact on health outcomes. In essence, the job of a health-care improver is to tune the system to generate good and consistent outcomes.

Second, we have come to recognize that, in general, one of the most effective and efficient ways to obtain better health outcomes is to design different types of systems to meet the differing needs of different types of patients. This approach has been described using business terms, such as "market segmentation followed by mass customization," which are mainstays of consumer-focused service sector design. In terms which might be more familiar to those in health care, it involves identifying major subpopulations served by a health system and then applying modern improvement methods (such as lean production methods, patient-experience based co-design, high reliability and safety science, and advanced health information systems) to design and refine a health-care system with the aim of producing the best desired outcomes at the lowest real cost.[5] By way of example, the Mayo Clinic in Rochester, Minnesota, has divided the primary care population that it serves into three subpopulations based on their chronic disease status (chronic complex, simple chronic and free from chronic problems) and is developing three different health-care delivery subsystems for each population.[27]

Improving Outcomes and Professional Development

When we turn to the relationship between improving outcomes and improving professional development, we are well served by reflecting on David Leach's dictum:

> Residents' direct participation in patient care makes it impossible to separate the quality of their experience from the quality of patient care. If patient care

> is shabby, their formation will be shabby; if it is excellent, they can learn excellence. Improving patient care improves resident formation.[28]

These words represent profound knowledge – often overlooked but thoroughly accurate. We all hope that health-care professional learners such as nurses and clinicians in training learn the best way to practice so that they can contribute to creating the best results for their patients. It makes sense, then, that the best conditions for good learning can be found in places where practitioners and staff work together to do the right things in the right ways to get the right results each and every time. This is a tall order and cannot always be achieved in the real world characterized by chance elements, uncertainty, and complexity. However, it underscores the point that the best learning is likely to occur in places that consistently track and measure their outcomes, benchmark them against the best-known results, and seek to continuously clarify the way in which good, reliable processes generate good, predictable outcomes.

One aspect of extraordinary learning environments that effectively develop the knowledge, skills, and values of health-care professionals is the consistent aim to attain the best possible results for individual patients and for the populations served. A key question in this kind of learning system goes beyond "what places do this best?" and asks "what is the theoretic limit to best outcomes?"[29]

It has been said that quality begins with the intention to make a superior thing. Consequently, intentional professional formation and development has a special opportunity in places that actually value and invest in an ongoing search for excellent outcomes. Another important link between good outcomes and good learning is found in the recognition of the need to incorporate practice-based learning and improvement into all clinical settings. The Accreditation Council for Graduate Medical Education and the American Board of Medical Specialties have recognized the critical role that practice-based learning and improvement plays in professional development and lifelong learning and have recognized this as a core competency that must be mastered by all physicians.[30,31] Professional formation and development will be strongest in places that pursue practice-based learning and improvement based on an ongoing attempt to link their own practice to the outcomes realized by the patients they care for.

Avoiding the Pitfalls of Being Too Focused on the Measures

A consistent theme in this chapter has been to promote the use of outcomes measurement as a cornerstone of improvement. Before concluding, we wish to call out some of the limitations related to measuring outcomes. It is possible to miss what matters most by focusing too much on measurement alone. Measures and metrics are at best surrogates of hoped-for results: the optimal level of health outcomes desired by the patient at the lowest cost. A few limitations of measurement are as follows.

- Measures that are intended to reflect a person's health status are not the same as the actual health status as experienced by that person. It is always necessary to attempt to understand how the individual views his or her own health state and what they hope to accomplish in order to enable an individual to make informed choices about treatment options in light of potential harms, benefits, and costs.
- There are times when specific goals for outcome measures may make sense for a population but run counter to providing good care for an individual. Lower levels of HgbA1c are associated with longer life and better health status and quality standards have been set to recognize the achievement of reducing HgbA1c levels to less than 7.0 among panels of diabetic patients. However, for a particular individual at a particular point in time the goal of lowering HgbA1c to less than 7.0 may not make sense. As an example, a primary care patient may be a diabetic with a HgbA1c of 7.5 as well as a smoker suffering from acute depression. Addressing the latter may need to take priority over reducing the HgbA1c at this particular point in time, but the patient's primary care practitioner will be, in part, judged on his or her ability to help that patient drop his HgbA1c to less than 7.0.

Just as it is important to not confuse the map for the territory, it is also important to not confuse the measure with what matters.[32]

Section 4: Conclusion

The point of health care, as mentioned at the beginning of this chapter and also a point in "the triangle," is to achieve the best health outcomes for patients and populations. It may help to recognize that people embark on health-care journeys that take them out of their homes and away from their jobs and into a complex health-care system. Patients hope that when their journey ends their health will be restored or that the damage to their health will be limited to the greatest extent possible at the lowest cost to themselves and their families. Tracking evolving health status over time and feeding that data both forward, as the patient receives care, and back to both the patient and the clinical team over time can produce better care for individual patients as well as create a rich data environment to enhance professional learning and improve care for future patients. Measures that reflect changes in health status (risk, disease, and function) can be used to design, implement, and improve health-care programs (innovative microsystems and mesosystems) for specific high-priority clinical populations, and, at the same time, promote patient activation as well as foster well-grounded professional growth and development.

References

1. www.dartmouth-hitchcock.org/about_dh/mission_vision_values.html (accessed June 26, 2012).
2. National Committee for Quality Assurance. *Report Cards*. Available at: www.ncqa.org/tabid/60/Default.aspx (accessed November 26, 2011).
3. Shneiderman B. Computer science: Science 2.0. *Science*. 2008; **319**(5868): 1349–50.
4. Nelson E, Fisher ES, Weinstein JN. A perspective on patient-centric, feed-forward "collaboratories". In: Institute of Medicine, editor. *Engineering a Learning Healthcare System: a look at the future; workshop summary*. Washington, DC: National Academies Press; 2011. pp. 149–70.
5. Nelson E, Batalden PB, Godfrey MG, *et al. Value by Design: developing clinical microsystems to achieve organizational excellence*. San Francisco, CA: Jossey-Bass; 2011.
6. Fisher E, McClellan MB, Bertko J, *et al.* Fostering accountable health care: moving forward in Medicare. *Health Aff (Millwood)*. 2009; **28**(2): w219–31.
7. McGinnis J, Foege WH. Actual causes of death in the United States. *JAMA*. 2003; **270**(18): 2207–12.
8. Weinstein J, Brown PW, Hanscom B, *et al.* Designing an ambulatory clinical practice for outcomes improvement: from vision to reality; the spine center at Dartmouth-Hitchcock, year one. *Qual Manag Health Care*. 2000; **8**(2): 1–20.
9. Mulley AJ. Personal communication; 2011.
10. Evans R, Stoddart GL. Producing health, consuming health care. *Soc Sci Med*. 1990; **31**(12): 1347–63.
11. Madans JH. The Budapest initiative: measuring population health status in surveys and censuses. The Joint UNECE/WHO/Eurostat Task Force on Measurement of Health Status, presented at the Eurostat Meeting on Disability Statistics. Dublin, Ireland, September 18, 2007.
12. Committee on Quality of Health Care in America, Institute of Medicine. *Crossing the Quality Chasm: a new health system for the 21st century*. Washington, DC: National Academies Press; 2001.
13. Nelson E, Mohr JJ, Batalden PB, *et al.* Improving health care, part 1: the clinical value compass. *Jt Comm J Qual Improv*. 1996; **22**(4): 243–58.
14. Hvitfeldt H, Carli C, Nelson EC, *et al.* Feed forward systems for patient participation and provider support. *Qual Manag Health Care*. 2009; **18**(4): 247–56.
15. Nelson E, Batalden PB, Huber TP, *et al.* Microsystems in health care, part 1: learning from high-performing front-line clinical units. *Jt Comm J Qual Improv*. 2002; **28**(9): 472–97.
16. Nelson E, Batalden PB, Homa K, *et al.* Data and measurement in clinical microsystems, part 2: creating a rich information environment. *Jt Comm J Qual Saf*. 2003; **29**(1): 5–15.
17. www.framinghamheartstudy.org/
18. Lim S, Murray C, Fisher ES, *et al.* Validation of a new predictive risk model for understanding the impact of the major modifiable risks of death. *JAMA*. 2011; under review.
19. Mausner J, Bahn AK. *Epidemiolgy: an introductory text*. Philadelphia, PA: WB Saunders Co; 1974.
20. Charlson M, Pompei P, Ales KL, *et al.* A new method of classifying prognostic comorbidity in longitudinal studies: development and validation. *J Chronic Dis*. 1987; **40**(5): 373–83.
21. Kazis L, Miller DR, Skinner KM, *et al.* Applications of methodologies of the veterans health

study in the VA healthcare system: conclusions and summary. *J Ambul Care Manage.* 2006; **29**(2): 182–8.

22. www.nihpromis.org/
23. www.dartmouthatlas.org
24. Centers for disease control and prevention. Reports from the National Medical Care Utilization and Expenditure Survey. Available at: www.cdc.gov/nchs/products/nmcues.htm (accessed November 27, 2011).
25. Reilly Associates. *WPAI General Information.* Available at: www.reillyassociates.net/WPAI_General.html (accessed November 27, 2011).
26. The Health Institute, Tufts Medical Center. *The Work Limitations Questionnaire (WLQ).* Boston, MA: Tufts Medical Center; 1998. Available at: http://160.109.101.132/icrhps/research/thi/wlq.asp (accessed July 24, 2012).
27. Nessee R. *Presented at the Intermountain Health Care Advanced Training Program (ATP) Alumni Reunion.* January 2011, Park City, Utah.
28. Leach DC. Using assessment for improvement: it begins with experience [executive director's column]. *ACGME Bulletin.* 2006; April: 4.
29. Krzykowski B. In a perfect world: interview with Paul O'Neill. *Qual Prog.* 2009; **42**: 32–7.
30. Accreditation Council for Graduate Medical Education. *Core Competencies.* Available at: www.acgme.org/acwebsite/RRC_280/280_corecomp.asp (accessed February 5, 2012).
31. Committee on the Health Professions Education Summit. *Health Professions Education: a bridge to quality.* Washington, DC: National Academies Press; 2003.
32. Korzybski A. A non-Aristotelian system and its necessity for rigour in mathematics and physics [reprint]. *Science and Sanity.* 1933; 747–61.

3

Better System Performance
Approaches to Improving Care by Addressing Different Levels of Systems

Mark E. Splaine, Jeremiah R. Brown, Craig N. Melin, Rosalind A. Lasky, Tina Foster, and Paul Batalden

Introduction

As has been described in Chapters 1 and 2, sustainable improvement in health care calls for a tripartite focus: better outcomes of care, better system performance, and better professional formation and development. In health care today, there are many pressures to improve system performance. Some of these pressures come from payers, regulators, accreditors, government, and other sources outside an organization. Responding to external pressures for improved performance in a reactive manner does not attract the long-lasting creative energies of professionals and is not sustainable. In this chapter, we illustrate an approach to improvement that recognizes the multitude of systems that are involved in the actual delivery of health care. We begin with the small systems in which patients and providers meet: the clinical microsystem. After describing what we mean by a "microsystem," we then provide three examples of system improvement. The examples provide insight into what it takes to make improvement at different system levels. In each example, we share both the "front story" – the overall results of improved system performance – and the "back story" – how this improvement happened, what was necessary to make it so, and what was learned as a result of this effort. We conclude the chapter by summarizing the elements from each example of better system performance related to the other two points of the triangle.

The Clinical Microsystem Framework
••

> *Every system is perfectly designed to get the results it gets.*
> —Paul Batalden, MD[1]

Nelson *et al.*[2] describe the clinical microsystem framework in detail in *Quality By Design*. This framework offers a patient-centered approach to understanding care in specific settings with an emphasis on the interdependencies involved and that multiple system levels are at work simultaneously and must be taken into account. The microsystem is the basic building block of the framework. A microsystem can be defined as the functional unit where the combination of a small group of people work together in a defined setting to provide care along with the individuals who receive that care. It has clinical and business aims, linked processes, a shared information environment and produces services and care that can be measured as performance outcomes. These living systems evolve over time and are usually embedded in larger systems or organizations. The meso-system represents a second level of system organization. Mesosystems combine two or more microsystems and can be seen in the functional journey of a patient through the system for an episode of care. Consider, for example, a patient who presents to the clinic with an acute complaint who then requires labs and X-ray and a return to the clinic for results, at which time a decision for admission is made. It is the mesosystem that will serve to connect the various microsystems the patient encounters, ideally assuring smooth handoffs and seamless care.

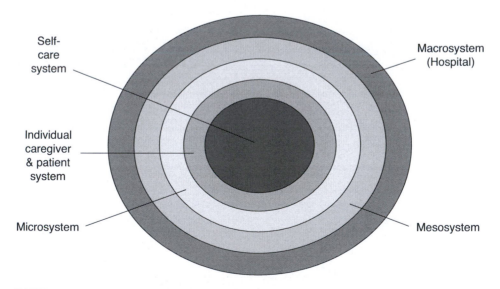

FIGURE 3.1 A multilevel systems framework for health care

A macrosystem is the larger organizational entity in which microsystems and mesosystems typically reside. Common examples of a macrosystem are a hospital or a multispecialty group practice. Figure 3.1 shows the relationship between the micro-, meso-, and macrosytem.

Case 1: Improving Care for People with Diabetes by Focusing on a Primary Care Microsystem

The 2010 US National Healthcare Quality Report's section on diabetes[3] notes the following facts about diabetes care:

- In 2007, 88% of adults diagnosed with diabetes had HbA1c measurement in the calendar year, 61% had dilated eye examination, and 66.5% had their feet checked. HbA1c measurement and foot examination have significantly decreased since 2002.
- The percentage of adults aged 40 or over with diagnosed diabetes who received three recommended services showed a significant decrease, from 43.2% in 2002 to 37.5% in 2007.
- In 2005–08, only 54.1% of adults aged 40 or over with diabetes had achieved control of their HbA1c level, 65.2% had their cholesterol under control, and 58.6% had their blood pressure under control.

Recognizing that similar gaps between what is theoretically possible and what regularly occurs in their local setting, the Section of General Internal Medicine (GIM) at Dartmouth-Hitchcock Medical Center (DHMC) began work to improve their systems of care for adults with diabetes in 2006. DHMC is an academic medical center and integrated health system that provides care to people living in northern, central, and western New Hampshire and eastern Vermont. DHMC is a multispecialty group practice with 33 different clinical sections providing care across the entire continuum. GIM provides primary care to 22 000 adults and averages over 50 000 visits annually. Patients diagnosed with either type I or type II diabetes comprise approximately 8% of GIM patients. Care for diabetic patients is provided by four different microsystems in GIM. Each microsystem includes a team composed of nurses, secretaries, physicians, physician assistants, and nurse practitioners. The microsystem also includes the patients served by that team and the information environment.

The Front Story: The Improvement

In 2006, a review of local patient care data revealed that only 18% and 39% of diabetic patients had had recommended foot and eye exams. Performance on glycosylated hemoglobin was at 88%. These results confirmed the judgment of the interprofessional leadership team of GIM that diabetes care could be improved. They realized the specific opportunity to improve diabetic care at the same time they recognized an opportunity to think more broadly about their systems of care for patients with chronic illness. A major issue for the team initially was the lack of regularly available data. They knew that their efforts to improve chronic illness care would be more sustainable, if they could build performance measurement into the work of daily clinical practice.[4] A first effort in this GIM improvement journey involved the leadership team working closely with the DHMC information systems staff to make web-based reports easily available at the level of individual providers and clinical sections, beginning with diabetes care measures. The GIM leadership understood that technical availability of the measures needed to be accompanied by methods for the integration of measurement within daily practice and training of health professionals in the use of the newly available data. The GIM leadership identified the role of a "health-care integrator" to help.

The health-care integrator became a key member of the multidisciplinary team charged with leading the improvement of diabetic care. The team analyzed the processes and professional roles of the clinical microsystem for diabetes care.[2] These observations led to several change ideas that the team tested over the following months, including:

- monitoring and displaying data over time
- detailed process understanding
- redesign of the role of the licensed nursing assistant
- design and implementation of a checklist.

The newly available data were displayed in ways that supported the improvement work, as shown in Tables 3.1 and 3.2 and Figure 3.2. Monthly reports were available for the performance of the microsystem team (Table 3.1) and for the individual provider (Table 3.2). The reports were ultimately color-coded (white, light gray, dark gray) to provide a visual cue to the emerging results.

TABLE 3.1 Diabetes Performance for Teams in General Internal Medicine

Diabetes Measure	Blue Team	Gold Team	Green Team	Orange Team
Diabetic patients (n)	310	366	377	231
Had HA1c in last 12 months	92%	91%	91%	86%
Had LDL in last 12 months	76%	79%	81%	74%
Had eye exam in last 12 months	68%	74%	69%	59%
Had PCP visit in last 12 months	95%	89%	91%	87%
Had microalbumin test in last 12 months	51%	63%	66%	64%

Diabetes Measure	Blue Team	Gold Team	Green Team	Orange Team
Had foot exam in last 12 months	71%	74%	73%	67%
Had pedal pulse exam in last 12 months	71%	73%	73%	66%
Had monofilament exam in last 12 months	70%	73%	73%	66%
Has had Pneumovax (ever)	82%	80%	80%	64%
Had influenza vaccine in last 12 months	61%	60%	59%	48%
Had BP check in last 12 months	94%	98%	97%	95%
HA1c in last 12 months greater than 9.0	8%	10%	10%	10%
LDL results in last 12 months greater than 130	9%	10%	11%	13%
BP in last 12 months less than 140/90	61%	62%	62%	65%
Flu assessment in last 12 months	63%	62%	63%	50%

Notes: White boxes are at goal; lighter shading is nearing goal; dark boxes indicate need for improvement. BP, blood pressure; LDL, low-density lipoprotein; PCP, primary care physician.

TABLE 3.2 Individual Provider Report for Diabetes Performance

Diabetes Measure	Individual Provider
Diabetic patients (n)	90
Had HA1c in last 12 months	93%
Had LDL in last 12 months	83%
Had eye exam in last 12 months	70%
Had PCP visit in last 12 months	94%
Had microalbumin test in last 12 months	70%
Had foot exam in last 12 months	77%
Had pedal pulse exam in last 12 months	77%
Had monofilament exam in last 12 months	77%
Has had Pneumovax (ever)	87%
Had influenza vaccine in last 12 months	71%
Had BP check in last 12 months	97%
HA1c in last 12 months greater than 9.0	11%
LDL results in last 12 months greater than 130	9%
BP in last 12 months less than 140/90	61%
Flu assessment in last 12 months	74%

Notes: White boxes are at goal; lighter shading is nearing goal; dark boxes indicate need for improvement. BP, blood pressure; LDL, low-density lipoprotein; PCP, primary care physician.

In addition, the monthly measures were displayed over time. Figure 3.2 provides an example of the measure "microalbumin screening." The results displayed on an individual's and moving range control chart show significant improvement in the rate of screening over time.[5] Monthly data points are shown, as well as the average performance (solid line) and the upper and lower control limits (dotted lines), which show the expected range of results given then-current system performance. Asterisks show where system performance improved significantly, allowing the control limits to be recalculated. The initial average performance was 36%. The average improved to 42% in August 2007 and 50% in October 2008. The arrows indicate the timing of the interventions: (A) training Licensed Nursing Assistants (LNAs) to monitor and inquire about microalbumin screening, to perform monofilament foot exams, and (B) to use an automated flow sheet as a checklist. As shown in Figure 3.2, performance continued to improve even after the second intervention, and the control limits narrowed, reflecting more reliable performance. Details of these interventions have been described elsewhere.[6] The improvement efforts have continued since this initial work. Further significant improvement has been made in microalbumin screening as well as rates of monofilament foot exams, patients receiving Pneumovax immunization, referral for retinal exams, and low-density lipoprotein cholesterol screening.

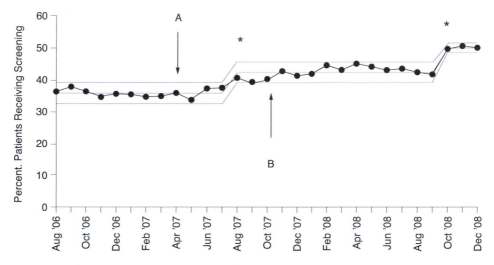

FIGURE 3.2 Control chart of results for microalbumin screening (the upward shifts in the mean marked by * indicate statistically significant improvements in performance)

The Back Story: Making the Improvement Happen

The improvement in the care of diabetic patients was promoted by many factors. First, the GIM leadership team supported and prioritized the work of the multidisciplinary improvement team. Second, the role of a health-care integrator – a clear champion for the improvement work of measurement development, staff training, and implementation of changes – was identified and a person was designated to fill this important focusing role. Third, the improvement efforts in GIM were connected to macrosystem level work on the improvement of diabetic care and other chronic conditions, resulting in shared insights about ways to redesign local patient care. Fourth, the display and regular use of data about better patient outcomes aggregated at the level of individual provider and at the functioning unit-levels of care allowed informed conversation among microsystem members and some "healthy competition" among teams. Fifth, the locally developed diabetes registry framework was quickly adapted and implemented for other chronic conditions, such as coronary artery disease and congestive heart failure. Sixth, the professional work roles of the LNAs were expanded to include use of the new data tools and monitoring the performance of the system. Before this project, LNAs brought patients into the exam room, obtained a weight and blood pressure reading and asked about the chief reason for the visit. As a group they were not very engaged in the care process, job satisfaction was low, and retention was a challenge. As a result of the role redefinition and new skills training, the LNAs are now empowered to oversee the successful achievement of agreed upon performance measures for patient care. Using the checklist and data tools developed in this effort, LNAs proactively prepare to address patient needs at every encounter. Job satisfaction is now high and retention is no longer a problem. Seventh, the development of the measures helped to formally integrate evidence-based care into the daily work and the regular data displays to the "real" levels of work offering participants actionable feedback on their care. Eighth, the use of data over time and statistical process control charts allowed participating health professionals to learn a new way of monitoring their performance. Ninth, by focusing on the actual processes and outcomes of care it became possible to better integrate resident learners into the care systems. Adopting common measurements for both faculty and resident clinic settings allowed recognition of need for comparable staff development (for the LNAs) in the resident clinic. Tenth, with demonstration of the benefit of these new ways of working for diabetic patient care, further changes in the organization of residency patient care

TABLE 3.3 Results for Selected Diabetes Measures, March 2010

Diabetes Measure	Blue Team	Gold Team	Green Team	Orange Team
Had microalbumin test in last 12 months	52%	68%	71%	67%
Had foot exam in last 12 months	69%	77%	77%	72%
Had BP check in last 12 months	94%	97%	98%	95%
LDL results in last 12 months less than 100	69%	63%	57%	62%
BP in last 12 months less than 140/90	59%	62%	63%	66%

Notes: Orange (resident) team results are now equivalent to results for other teams. BP, blood pressure; LDL, low-density lipoprotein.

(and their faculty supervision) became possible, bringing resident and faculty caregivers into the same clinical microsystem. As demonstrated in Figure 3.3, the GIM resident and faculty microsystem is indistinguishable in its performance compared with the other GIM microsystems without residents.

Case Conclusion

After focusing on understanding current performance, creating a system for regularly monitoring results, redefining certain health professional roles and offering additional training, and implementing improvements in patient flow, GIM markedly improved its care for patients with diabetes. The result was better system performance, health professionals working at higher levels and in more satisfying roles, and an enhanced sense of team function overall. These results included diabetes care and other chronic conditions as well.

Case 2: Improving Care for Patients with Coronary Artery Disease by Leveraging the Cardiac Catheterization Mesosystem

Better system performance can also be achieved by changes at both the micro- and mesosystem levels. The cardiac catheterization service, or "catheterization lab," functions as its own microsystem of care for an individual patient but also

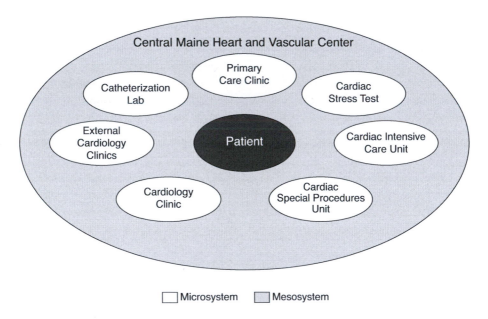

FIGURE 3.3 Multiple microsystems converge to meet an individual patient's needs within the mesosystem of cardiovascular care

operates as an intersection and integrating point for multiple other microsystems of care for patients: patient floors and holding areas, pharmacy, laboratory, medical records, and cardiology clinic to name a few (Figure 3.3). This example will focus on the reduction of contrast agent nephropathy, a priority of the National Quality Forum's patient safety work.[7]

Contrast nephropathy is a major complication following radiographic procedures using iodinated radiocontrast dye. Kidney injury resulting from contrast dye exposure occurs in approximately 10% or more of patients and costs an institution over $10 000 per occurrence from increased length of intensive care unit days and dialysis services.[8,9] Moreover, contrast nephropathy increases the risk of short- and long-term adverse events, including increased length of hospitalization, dialysis, and death.[8,10]

The Front Story: The Improvement

In 2009, the Northern New England Cardiovascular Disease Study Group adopted a goal of reducing the incidence of contrast nephropathy among its 10 participating centers.[10] A key component of this effort was understanding the five-fold variation in incidence across these centers, ranging from a low of 1.9% to a high of 10.1%. Site visits, structured focus groups and local process exploration was undertaken. These revealed marked differences between centers that had a uniform approach to prevention (mandatory protocols and use of prophylactic measures) compared with those that had a nonuniform approach (case-by-case model for prevention). The two centers with a uniform approach led the region with the lowest rates of contrast nephropathy. Both had developed and reliably used mandatory protocols to manage blood volume and to limit the duration of nil per os orders, allowing better patient self-hydration at home prior to the procedure. The remaining eight centers with a nonuniform approach had wide variation in the use of prophylactic measures such as circulating blood volume expansion. In contrast to the centers with lower rates of nephropathy, these centers more commonly restricted fluid intake prior to the procedure for a longer period of time (from 10 p.m. or midnight the night before) resulting in a higher likelihood that patients were volume depleted when they presented for the procedure. The full comparison of centers, data, and appendices can be viewed online.[11]

After sharing the data about the variation, participating centers explored the differences in their practices and began to redesign their systems of care to prevent contrast nephropathy. Illustrative of this improvement work was the response of the Central Maine Heart and Vascular Institute, an early adopter of change. Clinical champions from the center contacted the top-performing centers and discovered several possible local system improvements involving the cardiac catheterization mesosystem (i.e., the different microsystems and their interactions with the catheterization lab microsystem).

TABLE 3.4 System Improvements Undertaken at Central Maine Medical Center to Reduce Contrast-Induced Acute Kidney Injury

System Improvements for Contract Nephropathy
Involve a nephrologist
Evaluate contrast agent
Improve order sets
Flag high-risk patients
Simplify patient flow
Include system audits in rounding
Improve capture of the outcome

They began by reaching out to beyond their specialty and inviting a nephrologist to the catheterization lab sectional meeting. After identifying a need to change the contrast agent used in the catheterization lab, new contracts with a different supplier were negotiated and expectations of the pharmacy were revised; subsequently, the new contract for purchasing contrast went into effect for all radiocontrast services at the center. The electronic medical record was modified to incorporate standardized order sets, which would maximize volume expansion for scheduled patients. This required staff training and outreach to the referring cardiology practices that were writing orders for patients referred for a cardiac catheterization procedure. The electronic medical record was also used to create electronic flags for patients at high risk of developing contrast nephropathy. A new cardiac special procedures area was established to streamline same-day patients into the catheterization lab from a single unit as opposed to multiple outlying units. Physician assistants during rounds on post-catheterization patients were trained to specifically evaluate the patient for contrast nephropathy and establish maximum volume expansion to prevent kidney injury. Finally, efforts are now underway to monitor renal function up to 72 hours after the procedure using post-discharge order sets in patients at high risk for developing contrast nephropathy.

The Back Story: Making the Improvement Happen

The multiple system process changes described were important to the improvement of care, but they do not fully describe what was needed to address the complexity of successful improvement and better system performance. A first essential factor was the focus achieved by measuring and displaying patient-centered outcomes to bring a higher level of awareness of the situation. A "data wall" in the conference room showed recent outcomes for contrast nephropathy allowing every catheterization lab staff meeting to include discussion about contrast nephropathy. This awareness fed the interest in redesigning their care system and over three successive calendar quarters, they became the top-performing center in the region for contrast nephropathy.

Redesign efforts focused on standardizing care to prevent nephropathy. However, redesign would not have succeeded without an investment in health professional development. Mangers and staff were educated about clinical microsystems, coaching, and "Lean" to create a new culture of systems thinking and continuous quality improvement – making it the "new norm" to engage in changing their own work. In addition, a nurse leader was trained specifically as a microsystem coach to facilitate further improvement in the cardiac catheterization mesosystem (i.e., across all microsystems). Using this new knowledge, the team used its new process literacy to identify and address patient care delays in the catheterization lab. Establishing a six-bed dedicated cardiac special procedures unit for elective outpatients scheduled for cardiac catheterization standardized the process of patient flow to the catheterization lab. The staff in the new unit received the same competency-based training as staff from the catheterization lab and electrophysiology lab. Standard preadmission orders including hydration instructions, pre-procedure checklist, pre- and post-procedure patient teaching facilitated standardization of staff practices. Procedure delays, cancellations, and room turnover all improved with the establishment of a cardiac special procedures unit.

Case Conclusion

After focusing on reducing contrast nephropathy, instituting professional development, and implementing improvements in patient flow and the system of care for patients, Central Maine became the leading center in the region with the lowest rates of contrast nephropathy. The result was better system performance, lower rates of contrast nephropathy, and reduced system waste.

Case 3: Eliminating Hospital Acquired Infections in a Community Hospital by Incorporating a Macrosystem Perspective
• • • • • • • • • • • • • • •

Hospital-acquired *Clostridium difficile* infection remains a significant cause of morbidity and mortality.[12,13] There are many patient and system factors that contribute to *C. difficile* infection. The patient factors include advanced age, exposure to antibiotics, and immunosuppression. The system factors most commonly associated with *C. difficile* infection are insufficient hand hygiene, insufficient environmental cleanliness, and poor antibiotic stewardship.

Cooley Dickinson Hospital (CDH) is a 142-bed community hospital located in western Massachusetts. It has served the community for more than 125 years and has a voluntary medical staff of approximately 440 physicians, 1650 employees and approximately 10 000 inpatient admissions per year. Since 2004, the hospital's vision has been to become a model community hospital by delivering on exceptional standards for quality and safety; developing cutting-edge improvement knowledge (learning from others and developing new approaches); and teaching other community hospitals how to improve. Recently, it has decided to merge with Boston-based Massachusetts General Hospital.

CDH recognized in 2008 that *C. difficile* infection remained a persistent challenge (average of 0.82 infections per 1000 patient-days). As a result, CDH has taken a proactive approach in attempting to eliminate the problem of hospital-acquired *C. difficile* infection.

The Front Story: The Improvement

The Environmental Services microsystem work began in 2008 as part of a hospital-wide effort to improve care. In addition to members of the Environmental Services microsystem, this multidisciplinary team also included an infection control nurse and an administrative leader. After developing an understanding of their microsystem by studying the purpose, people, professionals, processes, and patterns, the Environmental Services microsystem team embarked on a series of improvement efforts. Together they redesigned the process for removing confidential trash and the removal of sharps; these efforts saved 6 hours of staff time per week. The team also focused on the number and storage of cleaning chemicals. By examining the types of products and specific needs for each they were able to reduce the chemicals used from 34 to 17.

Next, the microsystem team focused on the challenge of bed turnover. This was a problem affecting the hospital emergency department (ED) where patients often had long wait times to be admitted to the hospital ward. In addition, fewer beds were available in the ED for new patients. The initial turnover time for a bed averaged 65 minutes. The team observed that the process included many people, phone calls, and delays. As a result, the microsystem team implemented a pager system using existing technology for paging in the hospital and shifted from two people cleaning a room together to one person. This change resulted in a vastly more efficient system; turnover time decreased to 34 minutes. Interestingly, the new process was so efficient that staff were able to actually increase the time spent cleaning the room (from an average of 14 minutes to 24 minutes) while still reducing the overall turnover time. The new process had many benefits. Staff satisfaction improved among microsystem members as well as many people outside the microsystem (hospital nurse supervisors, transportation, ED coordinator, and staff nurses). Patients also appreciated the changes. The Press Ganey patient satisfaction survey results for cleanliness of the room and courtesy of staff rose from 50% and 58%, respectively, to 96% and 93%, respectively – a gain that has been sustained over time.

With the successes as outlined, the Environmental Services microsystem team looked to address additional problems. They were aware that the hospital-acquired *C. difficile* infections could be influenced by room cleanliness. They redesigned their room cleaning process from seven steps to ten steps, making certain that each cleaning included a dwell time for chemicals of at least 10 minutes (the time required by their cleaning agents to kill bacteria). They developed new and more vigorous approaches to cleaning rooms in which a patient with *C. difficile* had been hospitalized. However, none of these efforts made a significant impact on the hospital's *C. difficile* rate.

Undaunted, the microsystem team investigated other technologies that might be brought to bear on this problem. They identified a broad-spectrum ultraviolet light system based on evidence that it had been able to eradicate all major classes of microorganisms that cause hospital-acquired infections. This system was not widely used, but systems that used it, such as the M. D. Anderson Cancer Center in Texas and Cone Health System in North Carolina had reported great success. The microsystem team presented the idea for use of this technology to the hospital chief executive officer and the board of directors. They obtained approval and then worked with the company to pilot its use at CDH. Their initial pilot data was impressive. The hospital went more than 3 months without a *C. difficile* infection. Since the adoption of this technology CDH has had an 82% reduction in their *C. difficile* rates, and additional reductions in methicillin resistant *Staphylococcus aureus* and other infections.[14]

The Back Story: Making the Improvement Happen

The improvements made by the Environmental Services microsystem and the reduction in *C. difficile* infections achieved at CDH must be put in the context of system improvement at the hospital. The senior leadership at CDH has been committed to continuous improvement for many years. A detailed description of the macrosystem's approach to quality improvement has been published elsewhere.[15] We highlight a few of the key issues that contribute to its successes here.

Better Patient Outcomes

In this example, CDH targeted a specific patient outcome as a metric to monitor in their system performance related to hospital-acquired infections. This represents one of many areas in which CDH has improved patient outcomes. The hospital has produced a whole systems dashboard of measures that had been in use since 2005.[16] Whole systems measures are cascaded to unit specific measures throughout the organization to drive improvement. CDH has focused on improving individual patient outcomes by standardizing their practice and monitoring results over time in areas such as acute myocardial infarction, congestive heart failure, community-acquired pneumonia, and surgical infection prevention, all of which consistently have composite results in the range of 95%–100%.

Better Health Professional Development

CDH's investment in health professional development through educating managers and staff in the microsystems framework and training microsystems coaches dates to 2007. This effort involved a strategic partnership with The Dartmouth Institute for Health Policy and Clinical Practice to create onsite learning at CDH. The senior leadership team at CDH participated in these learning activities both as sponsors and as members of microsystem teams. It was because of these educational activities that the Environmental Service microsystem began the work highlighted. This approach to educating the entire hospital staff has helped to create a culture of systems thinking and continuous quality improvement at CDH.

Better System Performance

In implementing the use of the microsystem framework at CDH, there was an expectation that teams would improve many of the hospital's systems. The senior leaders asked microsystem teams to link their work to the hospital's strategic goals. However, the CDH leaders did not limit the focus of the microsystem teams to the strategic goals. They employed a strategy called "2 + 2 Charters" for each of the microsystem improvement teams.[15] This approach asked each team to address two of the hospital's strategic goals in their work and to identify two local goals that were important to their team. This strategy enabled the Environmental Services microsystem team to work on reducing the number of cleaning chemicals used and improving management of waste (team goals) as well as patient flow and hospital infections (hospital goals). As can be seen from the microsystem's improvement journey discussed here, the learning achieved by working on the team goals greatly informed and enhanced the team's ability to accomplish the hospital goals of improving system performance.

Case Conclusion

The focus of this case is on the efforts made by the Environmental Services microsystem to improve the cleanliness of patient rooms. In doing this work, this microsystem team discovered new and better ways of creating an optimally clean environment. They researched and obtained, based on their past work, a new device that uses ultraviolet light to sterilize all surfaces in a room. The new system has been implemented and the hospital *C. difficile* infection rate has dropped by 82%. This story highlights the critical role the macrosystem must play in establishing the context for and support of better system performance.

Conclusion
· · · · · · · · · · · · · · · ·

This chapter has focused on improving system performance. What ties these vignettes together and what anchors this "corner" of the triangle is the common commitment of knowledgeable people who want to work on the work of health care, not because someone asked them to but because they, like most professionals, want to do their best and to continually make their performance even better.

They recognized that health outcomes of quality, safety, and value are *caused*, they don't "just happen." They brought their gift of curiosity about the discovery of cause-effect relationships in the production of those outcomes in health care. At some level, they recognized that quality, safety, and value of care are all linked and grounded in the processes that come together to produce care and outcomes.

They learned that making the processes of work explicit – by making graphic representation of them and their interdependencies … by having conversations about them … by understanding their reliability and their variability – allows them together to "see" possible changes that could be designed and made to improve health-care system performance.

They learned that measurement can be a tool for learning, a means of discovering the variation that is present over time, but unwanted. They learned to study the variation and the causal systems producing it.

They have seen the benefit of constructing change theories that can be tested empirically, testing them, and then reflecting on what they have done.

In all this, they (and we) are acting on the insights of those modern pioneers – such as Nightingale,[17] Codman,[18] Lewis,[19] Shewhart,[20] Deming,[21] and Juran[22] – who decades ago offered counsel about the benefits of empirical and reflective work on work – applying scientific methods to the improvement of health care and the systems that create it.

In closing, we wish to highlight a few points. First, by examining the case examples, we hope the reader can clearly see how the link between system performance and better patient outcomes can be leveraged by embedding measurement in efforts to improve care. The case examples each illustrate the importance of data (often in the form of a registry) maintained by the macrosystem and made available to each microsystem. When coupled with a champion or person responsible for their use, data systems can enhance the monitoring of data over time as a core element in assessing changes related to system performance.

Second, professional development must be designed into efforts to improve system performance. Each case example has embedded in it efforts to develop the health professionals. In the case of DHMC GIM diabetes care, the focus was on enhancing training and role definition for nurses, as well as educating the entire microsystem on evidence-based measures and methods for monitoring and analyzing data over time. Central Maine Heart and Vascular Institute was able to achieve its reduction in acute kidney injury rates by activating a clinical champion, educating the microsystem team and developing a coach for improvement work to facilitate ongoing system improvement. CDH had adopted a program of training *all* hospital staff in the microsystem framework and rapid cycle improvement methods. This empowered the work of the environmental services microsystem, which ultimately led to the infection reduction.

Third is the importance of leadership in achieving system performance. Each case features leaders who promoted and facilitated improvement. In GIM, both the section-level leadership team and the health-care integrator played essential roles. The clinical champion at Central Maine as well as the nurse coach played critical roles in this site's ability to reduce kidney injury. The chief executive officer and chief operating officer at Cooley Dickinson as well as the manager of environmental services were the ones who guided the improvement in hospital-acquired infections. These leaders were responsible for leading at their assigned level of the system and were facile at connecting to and working with leaders at other levels of the system. These efforts help set the context for and facilitate the system performance.

In summary, we offer the microsystem framework as an approach to generating an understanding of system performance at multiple levels: micro-, meso-, and macrosystem. We believe that understanding one's own system can be used to promote organic, proactive system improvement – improvement that comes from inside the organization or system. We believe that this approach to improvement is likely more satisfying and sustainable than an approach that is driven from the outside-in by reacting to external forces.

Acknowledgments

We would like to thank the following groups for allowing us to share their stories of improvement:
- the members of the Section of General Internal Medicine at Dartmouth-Hitchcock Medical Center
- the staff at Central Maine Heart and Vascular Institute, specifically Susan Horton and William Phillips
- the members of the Environmental Service microsystem at Cooley Dickinson Hospital, specifically Daniel English and Linda Riley, as well as the many other health professionals there who contributed their improvement journey.

References

1. Carr S. *A Quotation With a Life of its Own*. Available at: www.psqh.com/julaug08/editor.html (accessed March 5, 2012).
2. Nelson EC, Batalden PB, Godfrey MM. *Quality By Design: a clinical microsystems approach*. San Francisco, CA: Jossey-Bass; 2007.
3. Agency for Healthcare and Quality. *National Healthcare Quality Report 2010*. Available at: www.ahrq.gov/qual/nhqr10/Chap2.htm#diabetes (accessed March 1, 2012).
4. Nelson EC, Splaine ME, Batalden PB, *et al*. Building measurement and data collection into medical practice. *Ann Intern Med*. 1998; **128**(6): 460–6.
5. Amin SG. Control charts 101: a guide to health care applications. *Qual Manag Health Care*. 2001; **9**(3): 1–28.
6. Lasky RA, Homa K, Splaine M. A quality improvement initiative to enhance the care of diabetic patients in a general medicine clinic. *Clin Diabetes*. 2010; **28**(3): 115–19.
7. National Quality Forum. *Safe Practices for Better Healthcare 2006 Update: a consensus report*. Washington, DC: National Quality Forum; 2007.
8. Chertow GM, Burdick E, Honour M, *et al*. Acute kidney injury, mortality, length of stay, and costs in hospitalized patients. *J Am Soc Nephrol*. 2005; **16**(11): 3365–70.
9. Subramanian S, Tumlin J, Bapat B, *et al*. Economic burden of contrast-induced nephropathy: implications for prevention strategies. *J Med Economics*. 2007; **10**(2): 119–34.
10. Brown JR, Malenka DJ, DeVries JT, *et al*. Transient and persistent renal dysfunction are predictors of survival after percutaneous coronary intervention: insights from the Dartmouth Dynamic Registry. *Catheter Cardiovasc Interv*. 2008; **72**(3): 347–54.
11. Brown JR, McCullough PA, Splaine ME, *et al*. How do centres begin the process to prevent contrast-induced acute kidney injury: a report from a new regional collaborative. *BMJ Qual Saf*. 2012; **21**(1): 54–62.
12. Kelly CP, LaMont JT. *Clostridium difficile*: more difficult than ever. *N Engl J Med*. 2008; **359**(18): 1932–40.
13. Oake N, Talijaard M, van Walraven C. The effect of hospital-acquired *Clostridium difficile* infection on in-hospital mortality. *Arch Intern Med*. 2010; **170**(20): 1804–10.
14. Trinchero C. *Using UV light, Cooley Dickinson Hospital Dramatically Reduces Infections, Provides Safer Care*. Press Release. Northampton, MA: Cooley Dickinson Hospital; November 7, 2011. Available at: www.cooley-dickinson.org/node/784 (accessed March 2, 2012).
15. Godfrey MM, Melin CN, Muething SE, *et al*. Clinical microsystems, part 3: transformation of two hospitals using microsystem, mesosystem, and macrosystem strategies. *Jt Comm J Qual Patient Saf*. 2008; **34**(10): 591–603.
16. Martin LA, Nelson EC, Lloyd RC, *et al*. *Whole System Measures*. IHI Innovation Series white paper. Cambridge, MA: Institute for Healthcare Improvement; 2007.
17. Nightingale F. *Notes on Nursing: what it is, and what it is not*. New York, NY: D Appleton; 1860.
18. Codman EA. *A Study in Hospital Efficiency: as demonstrated by the case report of the first five years of a private hospital*. 1917. Reprint. Oak Park, IL: Joint Commission on Accreditation of Healthcare Organizations; 1996.
19. Lewis CI. *Mind and the World Order: outline of a theory of knowledge*. 1929. Reprint. New York, NY: Dover; 1956.
20. Shewhart WA. *Economic Control of Quality of Manufactured Product*. New York, NY: Van Nostrand; 1931.
21. Deming WE. *Out of the Crisis*. Cambridge, MA: MIT Press; 1982.
22. Juran JM. *Quality Handbook*. New York, NY: McGraw-Hill; 1951.

4

Better Professional Development
Competence, Mastery, Pride, and Joy

Maren Batalden, David Leach, and Paul Batalden

This chapter took form as we reflected together and discovered connections between its substance and our unique individual experiences as physicians deeply but differently engaged in the improvement of health care. For clarity, we use our own first names and write in the first person in describing relevant personal experiences in the article. Making more generalizable sense of these individual experiences in the context of the chapter's larger themes, however, was a collective process.

Competence, for both individuals and communities, is a habit – a predisposition to good workmanship, reflection on experience, and the happy mixture of humility and hope necessary for forward progress. It is attentive to the outcomes of care and is nourished or starved by the systems of care. It is both a symptom of and a major contributor to the synergies of the triangle.

This chapter illuminates the triangle from the perspective of professional development. It is an organic perspective. If patient outcomes are the meal, and system performance the mishmash of cookbooks and utensils, health professional formation determines the quality of the cooks. Although professional development is about education, it is much more than education. It is more akin to professional formation – formation as in shaping – and it is not a compartmentalized activity limited to formal training programs. All who work in health care, from the housekeeper to the chair of the board, are being formed (and deformed) every day by both internal and external forces that lead to better individual and community competence and mastery or the reverse.

Much is known about competence and its development, and yet in many health systems it is the most neglected aspect of the triangle. Neglecting the formation of health professionals guarantees erosion of the quality of patient care, the quality of overall system performance, and the improvement and creativity of efforts to improve care, yet financial constraints and the pressures of time make it very easy to give it short shrift. Models of professional development are frequently either inadequate or impractical. G. K. Chesterton was once asked: "What one book would you like to have with you if you were stranded on a desert island?" His reply: "A Practical Guide to Shipbuilding" is relevant to our quest. Health care lacks "A Practical Guide to Health-Care Professional Formation" and instead struggles with profession-specific articles, books, regulations, and conversations about what might help. While all salute the importance of an interprofessional approach, few offer a comprehensive model for the development of all who work in health care.

The Competency Initiative

Paul's career took a turn into the professional domain of health-care improvement in 1985 when he was exposed to the work of W. Edwards Deming. Then a practicing primary care pediatrician, Paul remembers:

> As I thought about it, things had changed. When I started active clinical practice in 1975, it was not uncommon for patients to say "thank you" in some form at the conclusion of the visit time we had together. Ten years later, a visit in the same setting seemed to end with some form of the question, "Why?" What was the thinking behind my recommendations to patients and their families?

A new relationship of social accountability was emerging as the Samaritan and scientific technical traditions were now blending with newly empowered patients living in a world that expected and used more easily accessed and shared information.[1] Payers and regulators seemed to recognize and operate in this new world; health professionals felt uneasy. Joy and mastery in work seemed threatened.

The emerging quality movement seemed to offer an invitation into a new relationship with work for health-care professionals and a new framework for health-care leadership. Deming's paradigm – with its emphasis on designing for high quality rather than inspecting for poor quality, relentless and disciplined attention to solving problems within a "system of production and service," and the mandate to remove barriers that separate the worker from "his right of pride in workmanship" – seemed to chart simultaneous paths toward increased social accountability *and* a new professionalism.[2]

This path for health professionals would require new paradigms for health professional formation. Historically, professional formation for clinicians had been focused on clinical knowledge and its application to the care of an individual patient in the framework of a one-on-one relationship. In 1997 a regulatory agency formally broadened the mandate when the Accreditation Council for Graduate Medical Education (ACGME) introduced the six "core competencies" to guide the work of professional formation for physicians across residency programs.[3] In addition to the time-honored competencies of medical knowledge and patient care, the ACGME added interpersonal skills and communication, professionalism, practice-based learning and improvement, and systems-based practice. The role of the health professional, suggested the ACGME in naming these competencies, is not limited to the care of individual patients in one-on-one relationships. The six core competencies enlarge the scope of attention in medical education and ask the enterprise of health professional formation to produce more than traditional educational outcomes for clinicians. The Outcome Project, as the adaptation and spread of this core competency framework came to be known at the ACGME, began encouraging medical educators to be explicit about the connections between educational outcomes, patient care outcomes, and outcomes related to the performance of the health-care delivery system.

With its competency initiative, the ACGME opened a revolutionary conversation in health professional formation that linked undergraduate professional preparation with lifelong professional development and crossed interprofessional boundaries. In 1999, the American Board of Medical Specialties adopted the same six core competencies as a framework to guide their work with certification and maintenance of certification in the 24 medical specialties. In 2005, the nursing profession birthed the Quality and Safety Education for Nurses (QSEN) movement, which articulated a similar set of competencies for nursing professionals – patient-centered care, teamwork and collaboration, evidence-based practice, quality improvement, safety, and informatics. As with physicians, these nursing competencies widened the mandate for health professional formation and put health professional formation into an explicit relationship with patient outcomes and system performance.

The "motto" of the ACGME Competency Initiative, and in fact of the ACGME itself, became: "Good Learning for Good Health Care." Clinical work is a practical craft – a craft that uses art and science to effect purpose, to improve the health of patients and populations. The learning that is the focus of health professional training does not take place in the abstract. Health professional students are not learning for learning's sake, but rather they are learning to become more effective clinicians. The acquisition of these competencies is grounded in experience – the experiences of patients and experiences with the system in which care is delivered. It is not possible to learn how to be a good health professional in a setting that cannot deliver good patient care, nor is it possible to deliver good patient care or model good professional formation in a system that is not designed to support good patient care and good professional learning.

The triangle provides a conceptual framework for exploring this new paradigm in health professional formation.

But regulation such as the ACGME's competency framework can only do so much. Culture change requires that everyone in health care embrace these linkages and use them to make sense of their daily experiences.

Responsibility for Outcomes

Maren finished her formal training in internal medicine in 2004 as the new language of the six core competencies was beginning to percolate into the consciousness of graduate medical education. The relationships embedded in the triangle came to life after she had been working for about 6 years as a hospitalist in a public hospital.

Maren remembers:

> I was developing a growing sense of mastery in my work of caring for patients and teaching residents and students. I was getting a sufficient amount of positive feedback to believe I was doing a good job – occasional thank-you notes from grateful patients and families, a handful of teaching awards from learners, words of encouragement from supervisors in scheduled performance reviews. And then, at a retreat for physician leaders sponsored by the physicians' organization that employs me, I saw for the first time patient satisfaction data collected from patients discharged from the two inpatient medical units where I worked. I was shocked. Our report card from our patients about their experience of care suggested that our patients weren't satisfied with the care they were getting on our units. How could that be? I thought I was so good at my job!

The triangle reframes professional development – for all health-care professionals (from housekeepers to clinicians to board members) in relationship to patient outcomes – morbidity, mortality, the patients' subjective experience, and system performance. The triangle retraces professional boundaries for health-care professionals and invites us to consider the possibility that we are responsible for more than just our individual disciplines, intentions, and actions. Together with our patients and with other members of the health-care enterprise, the triangle suggests we share a responsibility for outcomes. It seems self-evident. Indeed, if not we health-care providers, then who? Though we habitually evaluate ourselves by reflecting on our individual intentions and actions, we know that outcomes matter. By our fruits, we acknowledge intuitively, we shall be known.

In the siloed bureaucracy of modern health-care institutions, health-care professionals often experience themselves as piece workers – covering over the weekend, arranging the discharge, mopping the floor, responding to a call light, following an order, interpreting a scan, copying a file. Accountability for patient outcomes is diffuse; any individual professional might reasonably feel that his or her professional obligation does not extend to outcomes. Neither our training nor our ongoing systems of performance evaluation have historically required us to think otherwise.

Maren reflects:

> In some ways, it seems like the implicit contract in my medical training was something like this: take a good history and physical, make an evidence-based evaluation and management plan, explain your thinking clearly to the patient and family and care team, listen and demonstrate compassion to the patient and family in front of you. I was, I thought, doing a credible job with that, as were all of my colleagues, it seemed to me. And we were all working really, really hard, putting in long hours and exhausting ourselves. What are we supposed to do when faced with evidence of poor outcomes for patients or poor system performance – unhappy comments from dissatisfied patients, rising rates of preventable infections, too much money spent?

If health-care professionals are – individually, collectively, and in partnership with patients – responsible for outcomes, we have a lot of work to do in restructuring health professional work. Clinicians need access to meaningful data about the outcomes of their work. Too often health-care institutions collect and report data in ways that don't inform frontline health-care teams about their own performance. Clinicians need real invitations (and genuine support from leaders) to participate in understanding and improving the processes that produce these outcomes that matter. The rhythm of work for most busy clinicians permits no time for shared reflection about the work and opportunities for bettering it. Clinicians need support for understanding the way in which outcomes are created by their interdependent relationships with one another and with patients and families. Despite the inextricable interdependence between clinicians in creating the patient experience, each clinical service line reports up its own hierarchy and approaches problem solving in discipline-specific ways. Clinical work is intrinsically service oriented; most professionals choose their work out of a deep desire to be helpful to others. Real change related to improving outcomes requires more than pay-for-performance schemes that add layers of extrinsic motivation to an already deeply motivated group of professionals.

New Relationships with One Another
· ·

Patient outcomes are produced not by individual providers but by the shared work of many professionals – both those at the clinical front line (physicians, nurses, nursing assistants, case managers, social workers, therapists, unit secretaries, housekeepers, and so forth) and those in supporting roles (information technology, medical records, radiology, phlebotomy, administrative leadership, financial management, and so forth). Shared accountability for patient outcomes requires new relationships among professionals. If our individual professional integrity is linked to the outcomes we are producing together, we have a new mandate for authentic, effective collaboration.

Maren reflects:

> My first epiphany was recognizing that my own professional obligation included some accountability for outcomes. My second epiphany was that I wasn't accountable alone. I was accountable as one of many; we were accountable together.

A traditional clinical practice environment isn't organized to facilitate shared accountability for outcomes. Certainly, the two medicine-surgery (med-surg) units where Maren worked as a hospitalist were not. Though nurses and doctors and therapists and social workers and case managers came together (with varying degrees of efficacy) to discuss care plans for individual patients, there was no forum in which people came together "on the balcony" to reflect on shared work and on opportunities to improve care processes. Using the tools provided in the workbooks developed by the Clinical Microsystems Group at Dartmouth,[4] Maren worked with the two nurse managers on the two med-surg units to create such a forum. A multidisciplinary group – a unit secretary, a nurse, a nursing assistant, a medical resident, a social worker, a case manager, a housekeeper, a physical therapist – began meeting for an hour once a week on each unit with the intent of building knowledge about their shared work and taking action to make improved outcomes for patients and staff and to improve system performance.

Although many in the group had actually been working together for more than 5 years, they actually had to start by learning each other's names. Meeting every week, the group has come to know one another and has grown in their appreciation for the contribution of each to the overall care of the patient.

Maren reflects:

> Although it is embarrassing to acknowledge, I now realize that something in my professional preparation and practice culture had conditioned me to see doctors and the doctor-patient relationship in "full color" while other staff

seemed to move about in "black and white." The doctor-patient relationship, I now realize I once believed, was the central business of health care. Somehow, through our weekly meetings, I began to see my colleagues in full color as if for the first time.

The recognition of this professional interdependence in producing outcomes for patients requires significant redesign. We health professionals train in discipline-specific silos with discipline-specific cultures and language. We hold discipline-specific assumptions about ourselves and about one another; we harbor discipline-specific suspicions. In health-care institutions, we hire, orient, evaluate, and provide continuing education for staff through discipline-specific processes. The deep hierarchy that governs relationships in health-care settings is powerful; it creates fear and inhibits trust. It is not surprising that we don't see our interdependence; every system is perfectly designed to get the results it gets. At the level of daily work within the clinical microsystem, we regularly make staffing decisions without regard to the implications for shared work. Each discipline uses its own logic for assigning patients, apportioning work, and determining shifts, which keeps us from seeing our interdependence and complicates our ability to form effective relationships. Even making time for frontline staff to meet with one another regularly across disciplines to have effective conversation about improving shared work is a disruptive proposal for many health-care work environments. The triangle provides a mandate for redesign that recognizes the importance of relationships of health-care providers to one another.

Beyond Work-Arounds

As every frontline health-care provider knows, getting clinical work done every day is complex. Every frontline health-care provider can tell stories of time-consuming paperwork that doesn't seem to add value, inexplicable delays and bottlenecks that slow down care, miscues and miscommunication, broken or misplaced equipment, frustrating rework, general policies and procedures mandating behaviors that don't make sense in a particular context.

Poor system performance consistently wastes resources of time, energy, and money and saps the creativity and commitment of engaged health professionals. Traditionally, health-care workers of every stripe are socialized to cope with dysfunctional systems rather than to master them. Even physicians, who occupy the highest rung on the historic hierarchy of power within the health-care delivery system complain about the conditions of their work and often seem to see themselves as "victims" – yanked about by the different mandates of too many third-party payers and external regulators, oppressed by productivity demands.

The dominant culture at the front line of many health-care delivery systems holds that in order to make the right thing happen for a patient, the patient-centered clinician may need to bend the rules, call in a favor, work overtime, take a short cut, create a parallel process. In their recent book, *Practical Wisdom*, Barry Schwartz and Ken Sharpe[5] describe the challenges posed by rule-bound bureaucracies (in education, law, banking, and medicine) upon professionals seeking to use their experience to make wise judgments. They praise "the canny outlaw" who stays faithful to his or her own commitment to do the right thing in the face of rules that mandate behavior that doesn't make moral sense. These "canny outlaws" abound in health care; the work-around is ubiquitous. But the posture of the canny outlaw is tentative as creating and sustaining work-arounds is exhausting (and ultimately wasteful.) Schwarz and Sharpe have even higher praise for the rare "system changer" who finds ways of employing his or her wisdom and experience in redesign to help in building systems that support professionals to do the right thing.

The triangle invites health professionals to be systems changers. Too often, health professionals encounter the quality improvement agenda in their workplace as a set of irritating, time-consuming, "one off" rules or protocols imposed upon their clinical endeavors from the outside. Improvement initiatives are born in a distant "c-suite" or a remote quality department and are experienced by frontline health professionals as "somebody else telling me how to do my job"; they are regarded therefore as the antithesis of encouragement for professional growth. In explicitly linking professional development and system performance, the triangle invites a new paradigm.

Maren's experience as a "system changer" on the medical-surgical units where she works is illustrative. Following the steps outlined by materials prepared by The Dartmouth Institute's Clinical Microsystem Academy, she and her colleagues began by articulating a shared purpose for their units. They built a new understanding of their unit by reviewing existing performance data together. They identified a focus for improvement – something small within their power to improve. They began running small rapid-cycle tests of change using a simple Plan-Do-Study-Act framework. Over the course of 2 years, they standardized the process of readying a room for a new patient. They hung whiteboards in patient rooms and helped all staff to develop the habit of using them. They introduced daily joint MD-RN bedside rounding, daily multidisciplinary discharge planning rounds, and intentional hourly rounding by nurses and nursing assistants. They created a formal two-step admission orders process with MD-RN "huddles" for each new admission to discuss care plans. They built new order sets for pain control and developed a new tool for patient centered pain assessment. They facilitated multidisciplinary workshops on communication skills, observed one another with patients and provided peer feedback. They sponsored multidisciplinary lunchtime conversations about unit-based culture. They created unit-based monthly service awards for staff and a satisfaction "exit interview" for patients on discharge.

Most of the initiatives went through several Plan-Do-Study-Act cycles. Some of these projects were altered so radically in the process of serial trials that the ultimate intervention bore little resemblance to the initial change idea. Some of these projects have given rise to good behaviors that have become incorporated as habitual new ways of work on the units; some new behaviors have been more difficult to hard-wire.

Maren reflects:

> Each step in this approach to making change poses its own challenges – identifying the right problem to work on, choosing a good change idea, finding practical ways of determining whether the change your efforts brought about is an improvement, coaching new behaviors effectively, building structures to ensure that the changed behaviors become habits ... But we have learned so much. It has been a real awakening for me to discover this sort of agency in my own work environment. One of my nurse colleagues in this work, Fran Huffman, may have said it best. When I asked her to describe her experience on our microsystem team, she said, "Together we imagine things that could be and we make them happen ... how great is that!"

In his best seller, *Drive: The Surprising Truth About What Motivates Us*, Daniel Pink[6] claims that old ways of thinking about human motivation – assumptions about carrots and sticks – no longer serve. The secret, he argues, to organizational high performance and personal satisfaction is understanding intrinsic motivation – the deeply human need to direct our own lives (autonomy), to learn and create new things (mastery), and to do better by ourselves and our world (a sense of purpose).

The triangle invites us to think about engaging professionals in the work of systems improvement in the spirit of Pink's framework – helping health professionals see patient outcomes and thereby reconnect with the purpose of their work; expecting them to build deep understanding of the systems in which they work and thereby develop true mastery in their working environments; giving them license to work together to reinvent the processes of their shared daily work and thereby direct their own professional lives. High-performing systems need health professionals to participate as change agents, employing all of their practical wisdom and exercising their rights and responsibilities to design effective processes of work that produce meaningful outcomes.

Two Jobs
• • • • • • • • • • • • • •

Professionals are recognized, in part, by their efforts to improve their own work.[7] Embedded in the triangle is an invitation to all health professionals to expand their understanding of their professional identities to include both *doing* and *improving* their work. Edgar Schein[8] describes the traditional culture clash in organizations between frontline workers (operators), middle managers and technocrats who design processes of work (engineers), and executives. Successful organizations, he argues, find a way to bridge the cultural divide among the three cultures, allowing operators to begin thinking like engineers. Leaders, who operate within a set of cultural assumptions of their own, are responsible for creating the conditions by which operators can learn to think like engineers and engineers like operators.

In the particular context of academic medical centers, it is worth noting the many ways this work resembles what others have called, "action research."

Action research has been defined as:

> An emergent inquiry process in which applied behavioral science knowledge is integrated with existing organizational knowledge and applied to solve real organizational problems. It is simultaneously concerned with bringing about change in organizations, in developing self-help competencies in organizational members and adding to scientific knowledge. Finally, it is an evolving process that is undertaken in a spirit of collaboration and co-inquiry.[9]

Action research begins with setting an objective. Recognition of a need to change and improve may arise from many sources. It proceeds by planning an action, taking the action and evaluating it – all grounded in knowledge of the work as process and system.

Coghlan and Brannick[10] have explored the challenges embedded in playing the dual roles of "improver" and "working professional." They note that in these dual roles, our work is informed by the need to manage our access to the relevant context and people as we attend to the real politics and ethics of change in familiar settings. Learning from and sharing our experience of improving care with others requires insight into how our "prior" knowledge has influenced – potentially enabling and constraining – the changes we have led. When properly attended to, helpful knowledge can be created and shared, even as real changes are made.

Patients as Partners
·······················

The relationship between professional formation and patient outcomes suggested by the triangle invites further reflection into the patient-provider relationship.

Health professionals don't offer patients a pound of healing, instead they offer a relationship that can help discern truths and enable more clarity about the particulars of what is wrong and what can be done about it; they offer a partnership that comforts and sometimes cures during the journey through illness. The "doctor knows best" approach of past generations is no longer appropriate; new models in which health care is a truly cooperative endeavor are emerging. Healthcare professionals, who have historically told patients what is going to happen, need to start inquiring into what patients would like – what values, preferences, and fears inform and motivate a patient. We need to be focused on outcomes that actually matter to patients and families. Health professionals need time for this kind of listening and courage to respond to what they learn by listening. It remains revolutionary in health care to design services that truly honor the values and preferences of patients and their families: designing patients' rooms to accommodate families; moving from fixed meal times to a room service model; allowing close family members into the operating room; letting patients read and enter information into their own charts; supporting and empowering patients and families toward greater independence in self-care at home.

Luke has cystic fibrosis. His mom, Kathy, works at the Dartmouth Institute as a research analyst on a project to improve the care of patients with cystic fibrosis. When Kathy developed breast cancer, she was well prepared to be an engaged patient. She meets every Friday with a group of "breast cancer conquerors." She reflects:

> The breast cancer care team knows us well because we are "engaged" patients. We actively research the latest treatments, learn from others' stories, and speak up for ourselves. When the breast cancer care team wanted to improve their care delivery and research informed decision making, they asked our group to participate. They asked us to help them map out the steps of care from diagnosis to 5-year follow-up. A researcher even went so far as to shadow one of our members from beginning to end, sitting through all of the chemotherapy sessions and making every radiation appointment. The team wanted to know if the care was timely, if information was clear, if it was easy to access, and if we felt comfortable and cared for. We also shared our issues with billing, insurance and filling prescriptions.
>
> I recall telling my oncologist that I had to wait over an hour for a scheduled injection on Saturday morning after my first round of chemotherapy. He asked me what happened; he had put in the order for the shot to be ready for 8 a.m.

I said, "You didn't happen to include the key to the cabinet in the order!" The nurse on duty had the order, but the drug was in a locked cabinet. Trying to find the person with the key took her some time. I know it was not her fault, but when you are feeling nauseated and exhausted, an hour can seem like a long time. I noticed that the waiting room was starting to fill up.

I knew many of this oncologist's patients opted to have chemotherapy on Fridays so as not to miss too much work. When I told him what happened and mentioned that the Friday clinic was staffed with only one nurse, he asked other patients and found out that delays were common on Friday. Armed with enough stories from his patients, he managed to find some help for this clinic. Problems with clinic wait time and missing keys were resolved. Sometimes it's the small things that patients mention that can change the whole experience of care.

If professional integrity – as the triangle suggests – is inextricably linked to patient outcomes and system performance, health professionals will need to learn different ways of being in relationship with patients. This learning starts with a new kind of humility for health professionals and a willingness to work together with patients as partners on system redesign.

Cultivating this sort of partnership with patients starts with small steps in our approach to ordinary, everyday work, as another personal story from Maren's experience illustrates:

I was supervising a fourth-year medical student who was performing an invasive procedure for the first time. The patient was a middle-aged man with end-stage liver disease whose failing liver led to regular accumulation of fluid in the abdomen. He had come to the hospital every 1–2 weeks for over a year to have the fluid drained from his abdomen through a large bore needle. "Don't worry," the patient said to the nervous medical student, "I can walk you through this. I've had it done a million times." "Perfect," I said. "I'll just stay here and watch to make sure everything goes well." I invited the patient into the role of teacher. He was masterful. "Okay, now pinch the skin and shake the pinched skin a little as you are injecting the lidocaine. It hurts less that way." As we sat waiting for fluid to drain slowly from his abdomen into five glass liter bottles, the patient told us about himself, his relationship to the alcohol that had led to his liver disease, his work teaching high school students about the dangers of substance abuse, his experiences in the health-care system.

It was, the student said, her best-ever experience learning to perform a procedure.

Making Promises and Seeking Forgiveness
··

The relationships diagrammed in this triangle invite the health professional to work together with others to take action that enables the healthy function of the health-care system and creates better health for people and populations. Using our individual and collective power to take action, posits twentieth-century philosopher Hannah Arendt, demands that we come to terms with irreversibility and unpredictability. In any complex interdependent social order (surely our contemporary health-care enterprise qualifies), human actions have consequences that we can never fully anticipate and that can never be undone. Therefore, Arendt argues, all human action requires promise making and forgiveness. The *Stanford Encyclopedia of Philosophy*[11] explains:

> Forgiving enables us to come to terms with the past and liberates us to some extent from the burden of irreversibility; promising allows us to face the future and to set some bounds to its unpredictability. As Arendt puts it: "Without being forgiven, released from the consequences of what we have done, our capacity to act would, as it were, be confined to one single deed from which we could never recover; we would remain the victims of its consequences forever." On the other hand, "without being bound to the fulfillment of promises, we would never be able to keep our identities; we would be condemned to wander helplessly and without direction."[12]

The relationships into which health professionals are called in this triangle require us to make promises and to seek forgiveness. We make promises to ourselves about how we will live and work in relation to our own core values. To make good promises to ourselves, we must be clear about our own core values and be honest in assessing ourselves. We make promises to our patients about our own performance, about the performance of the systems in which we work, and about our own roles in creating and maintaining those systems. To make good promises to patients, we must understand how well our system performs and what processes produce the experiences our patients will have. We make promises to our colleagues about our own contributions to the common work. To make good promises to our colleagues, we must know how our work is woven together with the work of others and how it connects to the purposes and actions of our organizations and the health-care enterprise in society.

More often than not, these promises are implicit. We discover them most often when we have failed to keep them. Explicit promise making invites a new level of accountability for professionals in relation to themselves, to one another, to patients, with the systems in which they work, and with the larger society. Creating opportunities to help health professionals explicitly seek and grant forgiveness in the context of the triangles of real professional work is the next frontier.

Reforming Health Professional Formation: The Next Steps

Creating a context with an ecology that nourishes personal and professional vitality invites work at many levels in academic health systems: governance, senior macrosystem leadership, mesosystems, and microsystems. Each level does different work. Each level offers the possibility of inquiry and action that can inform and support professional formation in the context of real health professional work.

Governance is the level of the health system that translates values into mission; that links institutional vision to social need and holds institutional leaders accountable for the quality, value, and safety of the work. It is at this level where the practice of noticing and measuring "what matters" can begin.

Some initial questions to guide inquiry and action at the level of the board:
- How can the board encourage commitment and investment on each of the three corners of the triangle? What metrics would help?
- How can the board encourage commitment and investment on each of the three "lines" connecting the triangle? What metrics would help?
- How can the board encourage the professional formation of senior leadership in relation to the other two corners on the triangle?
- What are the "important" things in this institution and how are they celebrated?
- How is organizational capability recognized and developed?
- What implicit promises have we made? What explicit promises should we make? How do we deal with promises that have not been kept?

The *macrosystem* is the level within a health system that translates institutional vision into strategy for improved quality, value, and safety; that models the desired culture of the work context and creates a shared institutional vocabulary; that outlines formal processes for leadership development; that authorizes and prioritizes work through building an infrastructure and allocating resources.

Some questions to guide action and inquiry for senior leaders within a macrosystem:
- What helps us stay connected to settings where patients and families meet the competency of the professionals who work in our organization?
- How do we help professionals grow and develop their capability?
- How do we help connect the work of all professionals within the organization to the sense of meaning and purpose that is embedded in the larger context, mission, and vision of the enterprise?

- How do we create a receptive environment for change and improvement?
- What support does the infrastructure of information technology and human resources offer health professionals for their work of design, delivery, and evaluation of health care?
- What implicit promises have we made? What explicit promises should we make? How do we deal with promises that have not been kept?

The *mesosystem* is the level within a health system that enables the work in support of patients' needs; that translates strategy into operating policies; that recognizes who must work together and actively works on the coordination of services and the collaboration across microsystems; that connects the "front office" with the "front line" and that actively fosters the development and leadership of the value-creating work of the microsystems.

Some questions to guide action and inquiry for leaders within a mesosystem:
- What do we do to develop knowledge of health care as a system, process?
- How do we enable an understanding of patient need and illness burden?
- How do we foster the measurement, display, and analysis of the variation found in the daily processes of health-care work?
- What helps us attract cooperation across health professional disciplinary traditions?
- How do we help those seeking to change and improve their work?
- What do we do to foster the linkage of "evidence" to the processes and systems found in the local context?
- How do we manage the "spaces" between the microsystems of care?
- How do we develop frontline leaders?
- What implicit promises have we made? What explicit promises should we make? How do we deal with promises that have not been kept?

The *microsystem* is the system level where patients, families, professionals from multiple disciplines, and information come together to reduce illness burden. It is the system level that translates policy into practice; the epicenter of "value adding" work for those served and for those serving. It is the microsystem that actually creates quality, safety, and value; that is the "sharp edge" where science and context meet; where most health professionals are being formed (and reformed or deformed) every day.

Some questions for leaders and professionals in the microsystem:
- What do we do to develop knowledge of our microsystem as a system?
- How do we understand our patients' needs and illness burden?
- How do we measure, display and analyze variation found in our daily processes of health-care work?
- What helps us to cooperate with professionals from multiple disciplines within

our microsystem and within other microsystems to make good outcomes for patients?

● How do we test and learn from changes for the improvement of our work?

● What implicit promises have we made? What explicit promises should we make? How do we deal with promises that have not been kept?

Conclusion

This chapter invites attention to one of the three linked aims: professional development. The inextricable linkage and interdependence of these aims – better outcomes, better system performance, and better professional development – means that failure or diminished performance in one affects and limits excellence in the others. The consequence of this truth requires that everyone working and learning in the system take Karl Weick's[13] counsel and develop an approach to their work explicitly attending to what they notice, how they make sense of what they notice, and how they take action – all of which needs to be framed by the entire triangle, not just their corner. It is in everyone's interest to help everyone else succeed. Learning how to discern and tell the larger truths that emerge from the larger system calls for relationship skills: integrity, civility, trust building, and abandonment of scapegoating as a mechanism for building social cohesion. Data needs to be shared and understood in order to provide the basis for good conversations about the work. Moving the linked aim of better professional development into the portfolio of "explicit" work in academic health-care centers requires the attention and creativity of all – leaders, professionals, patients, and communities. It will take health care to the next level, enabling pride and even joy to emerge in the workplace.

References

1. McDermott W. Medicine: the public's good and one's own. *Perspect Biol Med.* 1978; **21**(2): 167–87.
2. Deming WE. Japanese Methods for Productivity and Quality [seminar]. Atlanta: George Washington University Continuing Engineering Education; 1981.
3. Batalden P, Leach D, Swing S, *et al.* General competencies and accreditation in graduate medical education. *Health Aff.* 2002; **21**(5): 103–11.
4. Nelson E, Batalden P, Godfrey Marjorie, editors. *Quality By Design: a clinical microsystems approach.* San Francisco, CA: Jossey-Bass; 2007.
5. Schwartz B, Sharpe K. *Practical Wisdom: the right way to do the right thing.* New York, NY: Riverhead Books; 2010.
6. Pink D. *Drive: the surprising truth about what motivates us.* New York, NY: Riverhead Books; 2006.

7. Houle C. *Continuing learning in the professions.* London: Jossey-Bass; 1980.
8. Schein E. Three cultures of management: the key to organizational learning. *Sloan Management Review.* 1996; **38**(1): 9–20.
9. Shani A, Pasmore W. Organization inquiry: towards a new model of the action research process. In: Warrick D, editor. *Contemporary Organization Development: current thinking and applications.* Glenview, IL: Scott, Foresman; 1985. pp 438–48.
10. Coghlan D, Brannick T. *Doing Action Research in Your Own Organization.* 3rd ed. Thousand Oaks, CA: Sage; 2010.
11. D'Entreves M. Hannah Arendt. In: Zalta EN, editor. *The Stanford Encyclopedia of Philosophy.* Fall ed. 2008. Available at: http://plato.stanford.edu/archives/fall2008/entries/arendt/ (accessed February 2, 2012).
12. Arendt H. *The Human Condition.* Chicago: University of Chicago Press; 1959.
13. Weick KE. *Sensemaking in Organizations.* Thousand Oaks, CA: Sage; 1995.

5

Teaching the Triangle

The Dartmouth-Hitchcock Leadership Preventive Medicine Residency Program

Tina Foster, Stephen Liu, Kathryn B. Kirkland, and Paul Batalden

After years of thought and preparation, an idea for a new type of residency program was about to become a reality. Having anticipated the need to train physicians in the skills necessary for leading change to improve health care, a series of conversations with institutional and departmental leaders at Dartmouth-Hitchcock Medical Center (DHMC) and Concord Hospital (CH) and with accrediting and regulatory bodies were about to pay off: the Dartmouth-Hitchcock Leadership Preventive Medicine Residency (DHLPMR) program would be born. The mission was explicit:

> To attract and develop physicians capable of leading the change and improvement of the systems where people and health care meet. In conjunction with existing clinical residency and fellowship programs, participants' academic, applied leadership and practicum experiences in preventive medicine will focus on measuring outcomes and improving the technical, service, and cost excellence of care for patients and populations.

What would this look like? Who would want to join this program? Who would the faculty be? How would they guide the learners? How would the program understand the benefits to our residents and to the patients they serve? How would the work of the residents fit into the complexities of the medical center and hospital?

In this chapter, we will describe the DHLPMR program – its residents, faculty, and activities – and explore our deepening knowledge of the developmental journey our residents take, accompanied by their faculty coaches and the others with whom they work. We discuss how this journey reflects and deepens our understanding of the triangle, and how that framework can create sustainable improvements in care and the opportunity for joy while doing so.

This program would not have been possible without significant institutional support and the foresight of leaders at DHMC and CH. They anticipated the benefits for patients, for existing graduate medical education (GME) programs, and for faculty development that the program could bring. The program was uniquely privileged to have institutional leadership that deeply understood the need to create a very different type of learning experience in GME. As program leaders, it is our hope that we will continue to repay this investment by ongoing improvements in the value of the care DHMC and CH provide, the creation of new faculty who are familiar with all corners of the triangle and how they connect, and a deeper understanding of our regional systems of care. The program includes completion of the Master of Public Health degree at The Dartmouth Institute for Health Policy and Clinical Practice (formerly the Center for Evaluative Clinical Sciences), and culminates with a practicum experience in leading change at DHMC or CH. Residents also spend time in a governmental public health setting. Doing the combined residency generally adds two years to the total length of training, and residents continue to provide direct patient care in their specialties.

Since 2005, when the first graduate completed the program, we have graduated 31 residents who have combined training in preventive medicine with 17 different specialties and subspecialties. As these professionals have moved through the years of training, they have embodied the work of the triangle, and have provided us with new insights into what it takes to make these linked aims real. Small populations of patients defined by the residents have reaped the benefits of their work, systems of care have (often) sustained changes, and residents have experienced unique opportunities for professional development. But beyond the "intended" beneficiaries, we have found that faculty coaches and others associated with the program also experience renewal of their own energies and new insights into how to approach improvement challenges in their own settings.

> We began our work to create this program with a consideration of the competencies our graduates would need to work effectively in leading change to improve health care. Although all can be subsumed under the ACGME competencies of Patient Care, Medical Knowledge, Practice-Based Learning and Improvement, Interpersonal Skills and Communication, Professionalism, and Systems-Based Practice, we wanted to name specific skills not often referenced in GME.

Core competencies for our residents include:

- leadership – including design and redesign – of small systems in health care
- measurement of illness burden in individuals and populations
- measurement of the outcomes of health service interventions
- leadership of change for improvement of quality, value and safety of health care of individuals and of populations
- reflection on personal professional practice and linkage of that reflection to ongoing personal and professional development.

As a graduate medical specialty, preventive medicine embraces a diverse portfolio of medical activity, all of which include a focus on the health needs of populations, skill in measurement – of illness burden, risks and effects of interventions, understanding that professionals and those they serve come together in interdependent systems and awareness of the importance and content of the leader's role, and daily work making change and improvement.[1] This program embodies these themes and offers residents an opportunity to make them real in the daily work of care. So it made sense to seek formal accreditation as a preventive medicine training program. The DHLPMR treats each of these four themes in theory and application. Residents put these notions into practice, creating a personal portfolio of accomplishment to annotate their learning.

Who Are the Residents?

A medical student intending to pursue residency training in family medicine completed a summer elective in which he worked with several different family physicians in rural New England. He was struck by the variation he saw in how they addressed common problems. He witnessed the challenges they faced in trying to do their work every day. He knew he wanted to provide primary care in a rural setting. "Does it have to be this way?" he asked. He came to DHLPMR hoping to find a better way.

A common thread that attracts residents to the program is their frustration with a broken system that they have seen as new caregivers and that they know could be better; patient outcomes that are not as good as they could be; the often frustrating challenges of trying to provide seamless care; the demoralizing effects of "just getting by" day after day; and professional life lived in a world of workarounds. We attract residents who know that change in clinical care delivery has to happen at the frontline – the place where patients and the health systems meet; they seek knowledge about how to understand the way we deliver care and how to design and take action to improve it. Some see variation that appears unwarranted.

Others come with deep disquiet about the gaps between the evidence they know and the practice that they have seen: how can it be so hard to do the right thing? Some are moved by a specific patient experience. They bring curiosity, energy, and some important questions about how this program will invite them to spend 2 years of their lives.

Residents arrive as relatively mature trainees, usually having completed several years of graduate clinical training. This sometimes is accompanied by a bit of cynicism, and many are already comfortably ensconced in their own physician "silo." But they also bring a working knowledge of the daily care system's strengths and flaws, and a fundamental optimism that the system can be improved, along with a sense of the professional opportunity and obligation to improve that system. They come eager to "fix a problem," enthusiastic about the chance to develop new knowledge, and anxious about what appears to be a relatively unstructured path forward. They come willing but curious about what it will be like to be part of a residency that includes multiple medical specialties, and possibly paired with a faculty coach who is not of their same "species" of physician-specialty.

Thus, they arrive with a sense of the corners of the triangle – the need for better outcomes as they have seen in individual patients they cared for, the knowledge that a system of care in which they work can and must be improved, and a clear sense of their own need for greater joy and mastery as part of their continuing professional development. It is the program's job to grow the connections between the corners of the triangle, to broaden the understanding of what each corner encompasses, and to provide residents with experiences that inform their understanding of who "everyone" might include at the center of the triangle.

Who Are the Faculty?

We began our faculty development meetings in 2001, about a year before the first resident entered the program. At the first meeting, we announced the intention to refer to our core faculty as "coaches." We spent the next several months responding to feelings about the term, trying to elucidate what being a coach might actually mean, and crafting the language we would need to use to describe our faculty to others. As residents came to the program and our experience deepened, we developed a more complete image of the role of the coach, and coaches' meetings came to be run by coaches for coaches, creating that community of practice that was envisioned early on.

Our faculty coaches are likewise driven by a deep sense of responsibility to learners, patients, and society. In addition to recognition as excellent clinicians, many have completed the master's degree graduate program at The Dartmouth Institute for Health Policy and Clinical Practice (TDI), and all have a track record of leading change to improve care. In addition, we now have graduates of the program who serve as coaches. Additional criteria for coach selection include scholarly activity, ideally related to improving health care; organizational knowledge; demonstrated leadership skills; and effective communication and interpersonal skills. Our current coach guideline describes the role of the coach as follows: "A coach in the Dartmouth-Hitchcock Leadership Preventive Medicine (DHLPMR) program will guide, direct and counsel DHLPMR resident(s) in a transformative learning experience in leading change in care for a population of patients."[2] As discussed elsewhere in this volume, coaching is different from the usual work of faculty in a residency or fellowship program. Coaches may not know the answers, but they are good at asking critical questions. (*See* Chapter 7 for a more complete description of the faculty role as coach.)

What is the Work our Residents Do?

During the annual program retreat, residents and faculty coaches grappled with the question of how to describe and specify the work of the residency. Residents felt that what was in place was a bit skeletal – it needed more detail. How could we help the residents better understand the work before them? What questions would be most helpful for them to answer? What questions might be helpful for coaches to ask? The coaches and graduates in the room knew every resident follows a slightly different path – the general guidelines that were developed when we started the program were not quite enough. All knew the reflective component was key, but sometimes hard to capture. A group convened to explore the lived experience of recent graduates, and to use that experience to provide a guideline for incoming trainees – what is the common path that most residents follow? When, along the way, should important questions be raised? How do these relate to our program objectives and residency requirements?

Residents spend the first year in DHLPMR developing an understanding of a patient population of interest and exploring ways that population's outcomes might be improved. They often arrive with an idea of what they want to work on, informed by their prior experiences in residency or fellowship. Their exploration and further definition of the patient population is enhanced by their Master in Public Health graduate coursework, where they have the opportunity to explore the evidence related to optimal care, to understand current processes of care, and to work with data reflecting current outcomes. We require that residents present their plans in an early formative and later in a summative report to our Practicum

Review Board (PRB), which approves all resident practicum plans. Chaired by senior leadership of the medical center, the PRB includes physician, nursing, and administrative leaders. The "resident-eye view" of care often includes some surprising and compelling stories, as residents work to take institutional priorities and match them with real patient experiences. In the second year of the program, residents work with the teams they have assembled to make their proposed changes a reality. Inevitably, the best-laid practicum plans are altered and revised, and the final product rarely looks exactly like the initial proposal; it is navigating these waters of uncertainty, using small tests of change and an unrelenting focus on the global and specific aims that produces the transformation from passive observer to engaged leader in our learners, and in those who work with them.

> The group met over several months, and developed a document that describes the general work of the program in detail; residents are advised to work with the coaches to use this as a map or guide to the territory they are entering. It was christened the "Developmental Journey."

Here, we present key steps of the journey and some illustrative stories. A current version of the developmental journey in its entirety is shown in Table 5.1. We present this as our current residents use it, but we know that it is a living document and will be continually revised to better suit their needs. We feel that this description of tasks and questions facing one embarking on leading significant change within clinical microsystems may be useful to others, and that in addition to specifying aspects of outcomes and system performance to be considered, the reflective prompts will spur ongoing professional development. In the next few sections we highlight selected steps along this developmental journey. We indicate the major topics raised during selected steps, but encourage readers to review the full document to see the complete set of topics, sub-questions posed, and, importantly, relevant questions for faculty coaches.

Describe a patient case where a patient received care that was less than ideal, unsafe, or led to a poor outcome

An Infectious Disease Fellow recalls a patient with severe sepsis whose first dose of potentially life-saving antibiotics was not given for over 12 hours after it was ordered. How often does this happen, she wondered? After wrestling with what matters (first dose of antibiotics for patients with sepsis? first dose of "stat" antibiotics?), she elects to learn more about the timing of first-dose antibiotic administration, and discovers that the mean time from ordering to administration is over 4 hours – perhaps not surprising to the harried nurses on the floor, but shocking to the physicians. As she builds understanding about where the delays occur, she encounters a sea of pointing fingers. The floor nurses report that pharmacy turnaround time is slow; the pharmacy says orders take too long to arrive from the floor. Analysis of the actual timing of events shows that the longest delays occur from the time an antibiotic is released from the pharmacy until it is infused. This requires exploration of the geography of the unit she is working in, and careful attention to the actual processes of medication ordering and administration. Along the way, she uncovers trays of unused antibiotics returned to the pharmacy every morning to be discarded, wasted because they were duplicates, medications that were thought to have never arrived on the floor, and were thus re-ordered.

In our experience, residents often find a particular case that triggers their interest in a specific population, or a story that is especially emblematic of the problem they wish to address. These patient stories are compelling for others to hear, and create a grounding reality around which teams can convene. The case also offers a starting point for exploration of the actual patient experience, and begins to ask questions about current system performance. It is often a helpful starting place when residents begin to describe their work to others. The coaching questions speak to the personal link and professional development of the resident, and seek to begin to link this individual event to a broader understanding of how care is provided.

Current knowledge and evidence base: provide a summary/ comprehensive review of the current knowledge of the care problem being addressed

A Rheumatology fellow in the program knows that access to the clinic is a problem. Importantly, there is good evidence that it is crucial for long-term outcomes: patients with rheumatoid arthritis will have higher remission rates if treated within 12 weeks of the onset of symptoms.

The academic learning in the early part of the first year of the program includes the opportunity to conduct a systematic review or meta-analysis of the peer-reviewed literature. Many residents complete their reviews as related to their population of interest. Even though some do not complete a formal review of this nature for their population, all begin trying to understand the best science and the best evidence available.

Local context: learn about the patient population in your local setting that includes the described patient case

A resident explores the clinical microsystem that provides care for pregnant women. Her conversations with team members explore the differences between how midwives, residents, and attending physicians approach the topic of HIV screening with their patients. A close examination of the process of discussing and ordering labs illuminates the barriers to "opt-out" screening.

It is here that residents often begin to convene their team and learn from a variety of perspectives what care entails. They begin to better understand the experiences and outcomes of a small population of patients; they begin to define and describe the clinical microsystems that participate in the care, and they engage with the clinicians and staff involved in that care. New ways of learning about patients and families are explored. This is often the first time that residents have formally considered outcomes for a small population of patients, rather than general impressions gained from their care for a series of individual patients. It is often their first experience trying to describe the systems of care, and their first opportunity to observe and graphically depict the processes and variation within those systems. It is often their first experience with hearing from a variety of perspectives about what care entails, and their first foray into the institution's "data warehouse."

Local context: define the local care problem or care gap

A Fellow in infectious disease wants to work on improving hand hygiene. He reviews results on different units, and ultimately decides to work on the unit with the lowest locally reported rates of hand hygiene. He has educational strategies, surveys, and other interventions in mind. However, it is not until he spends time watching how the work is done that he begins to see a reasonable strategy for intervention.

Although residents often start the program with a sense of the population they are interested in (and many times with a solution designed in advance – a common pitfall in responding to care gaps), we encourage them to delve more deeply into what the actual problem is, and what factors might contribute to the results currently obtained. This often requires new ways of looking at things, new ways of learning about actual processes, and a good deal of work to learn what data is available, as well as what data would be desirable.

System dysfunctions begin to seem clearer, and residents begin to gain insight into who will be needed at the table as the hard work of changing the system gets underway. The coaching questions serve to help ground them in current reality, and invite them to experience the problem in new ways, building on others' perspectives.

Develop an improvement team

Nursing leadership on the inpatient medical unit is in agreement with a proposed intervention to reduce hospital readmissions. The work is progressing and the group is meeting regularly. The resident struggles with how much to direct, and how much to let the group design its own work. He struggles even more when some key group members accept an early retirement offer.

Finding willing team members is often easy, especially as many members of the care team share the residents' frustrations about outcomes and systems. However, actually getting those team members together, leading productive meetings, and understanding the local politics of change are huge areas of learning for our residents. Although many residents are comfortable with the role of team leader in clinical care, this is very different. They are exposed to a variety of perspectives and learn about how the system works in a very new way. As they do this work with the team, they encounter the realities of work in a complex organization – for example, people changing jobs, people reprioritizing the work in response to other, competing initiatives. It is often here that a sense of what professional development means for *everyone* begins to develop – the team members must see the benefit for patients and their own work, but must also be able to stretch themselves and develop their own skills, as well as help the resident develop his or her own.

Identify and define measures that can be used to assess the quality of care, based on your knowledge of the current evidence, local context, and patient population

A medicine-psychiatry resident is working to improve utilization of the Psychiatric Partial Hospitalization Program (PPHP), an intensive outpatient alternative to hospitalization. In the regular work-rounds session, where residents and faculty discuss work in progress, he is challenged to explain how the value of the PPHP can be demonstrated – what are the patient-centered outcomes? Some months later, he returns with data to show that on a validated scale of depression and anxiety, most patients are leaving the PPHP with improvements in their scores, and none have worsened. In addition, he can show how utilization of the program has increased, and is beginning to collect information that will show improved access to needed inpatient beds as patients eligible for PPHP are directed there.

Getting measurement "right" is crucial for the work, and is always a challenging step. Residents find themselves confronted with a variety of data sources, some reliable and some not, and often need to define additional data that the team will need to collect. The discipline of creating operational definitions is necessary, but is a skill that takes time and practice. As DHMC transitioned to a new electronic health record (*see* Chapter 6), these issues became even more challenging, but also provided residents an opportunity to see ways to work to build a better system and engage with information systems leadership. But beyond data systems, there are needs to understand what lies "under" the metrics, and how measures that are patient-centered can be developed. How can everyone (including patients) become part of the team?

Begin to define intervention(s) that could improve care for your patient population, based on your knowledge of the current evidence, local context, care processes, and patient population

Another psychiatry resident enters the program after completing two years of her training in psychiatry. She has an interest in oncology, and in her conversations with others, she learns of the gap between the mental health needs of patients seen in the head and neck cancer clinic and the resources available. Entry to this microsystem, which is not one with which she is familiar, is eased by her shared course work with the ENT section chief (a fellow student in the master's degree program at TDI) and the support of the primary head and neck oncologist, who is also the hematology/oncology fellowship program director. As she further explores the microsystem for interest in this area, she learns that the social worker assigned to this area is familiar with many support resources through her work with the Comprehensive Breast Program. She adapts evidence-based screening tools for distress and pilots their use in the microsystem, and works with the clinicians to develop an algorithm supporting their treatment and referral decisions for patients who are found to be distressed. All become aware of a wealth of resources available that were previously untapped. Other microsystems within the cancer center express interest, and her work begins to spread.

As noted earlier, sometimes new information must be collected. Residents have to explore, understand, and test the care processes in the clinical setting, but it can be very hard to make small tests of change in systems where rewriting a policy or designing an elaborate "fix" is the norm. Communicating to the team that many small experiments will be run and that the ideas will evolve over time can be hard. Similarly, working in an academic health center with clinicians skilled in traditional research methods can be challenging – how can it be acceptable to deviate from the "protocol"? Our residents regularly confront in themselves the rush to a solution, the desire to solve the problem before it is understood. They learn the value of trying something, revising it, and trying again. And as they do this, the team learns with them. Similarly, in a medical culture where a scarcity mentality often predominates, and where we are used to complaining about "the system," the discovery of new resources, or resources that were already in place but untapped, can generate a new sense of engagement. Developing appreciative inquiry skills[3] is another important aspect of the training.

Understand the methods that will be used to measure the impact of the intervention on the patient population; consider the display and analysis of measures

A pathology resident has worked to decrease errors in specimen labeling in the emergency department. Although the lab is used to thinking about the thousands of specimens they receive each day, the data she has to feed back to the microsystem doesn't seem helpful. They currently receive information on errors per month, but the number seems very small and not actionable. It's hard to imagine what it really means in terms of daily work. Working with the program's improvement specialist, she develops a way to present this information as errors per day, and it becomes clear that mislabeled specimens arrive from the unit every few days. This ability to see the data differently, coupled with stories of the rework, frustration, patient discomfort, and potential for real harm created by mislabeling created space for discussion and assessment of the effects of improvement efforts.

A key faculty member, added shortly after the program began, is our improvement specialist. With expertise in both quantitative and qualitative analysis, she works alongside faculty coaches and residents to explore the best ways to analyze and understand the data collected. Residents also have access to experts in measurement through their coursework, and sometimes in the local settings where they are working. As they do this work, they are constantly challenged to understand measurement for improvement, which often differs from the measurement for research that is familiar from prior medical training.

Interpretation of results: describe the results of the implementation of the intervention and explore the limitations

A resident works to improve the care for patients with community-acquired pneumonia. As measures related to this condition are publicly reported, there is intense interest in how his work has affected care. But he can also see how the system within which he is working both potentiated and challenged his work, and he explores this in the context of complexity theory and Glouberman and Zimmerman's[4] thinking on simple, complicated, and complex problems. Ultimately he publishes this work with others from the clinical microsystem and residency program, not simply as an example of how care for pneumonia was improved, but as a scholarly exploration of how problems must be understood in order to develop appropriate solutions.[5]

As a program focused on learning for all – not just residents but also faculty, microsystem members, and the institution – understanding and interpreting the results of the practicum is integral to the work. This may require exploration of new paradigms and ways of thinking, and creative ways to share them. Describing the patient outcomes may be relatively simple when compared to understanding how a specific setting influenced the results. How can the learning from one microsystem benefit others? How can the mesosystem and macrosystem learn as well? The residency regularly convenes faculty and residents to consider the work of scholarly writing about improvement. Using the SQUIRE guidelines[6] as our primary framework, we share work in progress, and consider how to best describe the important details of a specific setting and results, while simultaneously attempting to understand what might be useful for others. This clearly calls on all corners of the triangle at once – how can we link outcomes in a particular setting to knowledge about a larger set of systems in a way that can be applied in other settings as well?

Reflect on successes and difficulties in implementing the improvement interventions: How will you plan for sustainability? What are the lessons learned?

A resident considers her next steps. She has worked hard to develop a new way of thinking about care for complex patients in her clinic, and has successfully modified the electronic record to facilitate their use. The number of patients with care plans has increased, and information important to patients as well as providers is now readily available and regularly updated. She is graduating, and will be moving to another institution where care plans have not been used. How can she leverage her new skills and insights in her new work setting? How will she continue to work on something that is now of great importance to her? As she moves into her new position, she is able to work with the group preparing for the implementation of a new electronic record to develop and deploy a care plan. Some of the issues are similar, others are new, but she feels confident in her ability to build on her experience as a resident in leading this change.

We regularly celebrate our residents' successes, and sometimes mourn changes that were not sustained. We must often remind ourselves that as this is a training program, the ultimate measure of success is the learning that occurs; not how much the needle of change moves. At times, a practicum that does not produce major improvements in care might be a much more valuable experience than one in which care was clearly improved, but where the resident did not have the opportunity to lead and learn from leading. Thus, our final resident presentation to the Practicum Review Board focuses not only on results, though these are clearly important. The highlight of the presentation is the discussion of the lessons learned, for the individual and the system. These are the lessons that residents will carry with them as they move to the next stages of their careers. While residents leave with a new set of "tools" related to process analysis and measurement, it is their ability to describe their leadership experience, to convene an interprofessional team, and to continually reflect on what they have done that characterizes their accomplishments and authenticates their work for future employers.

The Developmental Journey
· ·

It is important to note that, like many journeys, this one is not linear. Steps occur simultaneously and are repeated; some are deferred. A single step labeled "intervention" could convey the impression that there is one major intervention, as opposed to a series of small tests of change, which sometimes result in an overall intervention that is rather different than the original plan outlined by the resident to the Practicum Review Board. Recall that real improvement and change in complex social systems is a reflexive phenomenon – working on a change changes the context. Some questions may be more important than others for specific small tests of change. However, the primary benefit of this explicit design of the path residents are likely to follow is its ability to stimulate good conversation between coach and resident, to alert residents to nuances of thinking about better outcomes and better system performance, and to further identify ways in which everyone can continue to develop and grow in their work. We know that we will continue to revise and refine this document over the next few years. As with its creation, input for its continuing revision will include all members of our residency community. For use in the residency, we have matched program-specific goals and objectives and created assessment tools which reflect those goals. These as well will require refinement over time.

We are pleased to share our early formulation of the developmental journey here as it represents the lived experiences of residents, coaches, and interdisciplinary teams who have successfully planned and led improvement, and we hope that it can suggest ways to make the triangle come to life in a variety of settings. We are constantly reminded in our program of the power of close attention and observation, of the unique view of care in an academic setting that residents have, and of the tremendous energy and ability they can bring to efforts to improve care.

TABLE 5.1 Dartmouth-Hitchcock Leadership Preventive Medicine Residency Program Developmental Journey, 2011

Resident Work and Questions for Consideration	Goals and Objectives (ACGME Core Competencies in Capital Letters)[6]	Questions Faculty Might Ask
Patient Case		
1. Describe a patient case where a patient received care that was less than ideal, unsafe, or led to a poor outcome. a. Why is this case important to you? b. Why is this important to the institution, local community and/or nationally? c. What factors and care processes contributed to the poor care received?	Apply knowledge and skills to learning about illness burden of individuals in populations (MK, PC, PBLI, SBP)	Why is this particular case important to you? How were you able to understand the patient's and family's experience?

Resident Work and Questions for Consideration	Goals and Objectives (ACGME Core Competencies in Capital Letters)[6]	Questions Faculty Might Ask
Patient Case (*cont.*)		

d. Who was involved with caring for the patient?
  i. Care setting
  ii. Care providers
  iii. Patient and family considerations
  iv. Consider use of a fishbone diagram
e. What specific outcomes or process measures could quantify the care received?
f. Is there current literature or guidelines that could provide guidance on the ideal care that was or wasn't provided?
	Identify the ABNA using available metrics and standard of care (PC, MK, PBLI, SBP)
	Describe/model a clinical microsystem (SBP)
	Describe current processes of care (PC, SBP)
	Participate in identifying system errors and implementing potential systems solutions (SBP)
		Why is this situation important here, now?
		Can you draw the general overview of the process of care?
		What sources of information did you use?
		Who else will think this is an important problem?

Current Knowledge and Evidence Base		

2. Summary/comprehensive review of the current knowledge of the care problem being addressed.
a. Are there national guidelines and recommendations for ideal care?
b. What are the clinical studies documenting the improvement in outcomes with patient populations with certain medical interventions?
c. What does the literature say about the difficulties and barriers with implementing evidence into actual care settings?
d. Are there quality improvement reports from institutions that have attempted to improve the care problem?
e. What is your critical appraisal of literature that considers possible bias, confounding, study design, and/or funding sources that could affect the stated conclusions and/or generalizability?
f. What are the process and outcome quality measures associated with the care problem?
  i. Publicly reported
  ii. CMS/JCAHO measures
  iii. NQF
	Conduct a literature review (MK, PBLI)
	Critically appraise and synthesize available scientific evidence that contributes to the quality of care for defined population (MK, PBLI)
	Evaluate relevance of literature to a given population (MK, PBLI, PC)
	Locate, appraise, and assimilate evidence from scientific studies related to patients' health problems (PBLI)
	Use computers for reference retrieval, statistical analysis, graphic display, database management, and communications (PBLI)
	(Select appropriate evidence-based clinical preventive services for individuals and populations [PC])
		How did you identify important studies?
		What sources were used to complete the review?
		What did you specifically *not* include and why?
		What was missing from the literature?

Local Context: Patient Population and Care Processes		
3. Learn about the patient population in your local setting that includes the described patient case.	Define and describe a patient population (PC, PBLI)	What is the best way to access the data for this system?

(continued)

Resident Work and Questions for Consideration	Goals and Objectives (ACGME Core Competencies in Capital Letters)[6]	Questions Faculty Might Ask
Local Context: Patient Population and Care Processes (*cont.*)		

4. What are the demographics of your patient population?
5. How many such patients are there?
6. What is the illness burden of the population?
  a. Number of comorbidities
  b. Average LOS
  c. Number of medications
  d. Functional status
  e. Health care utilization – number of hospitalizations, clinic visits, ED visits
7. Where are the patients seen?
  a. Inpatient, outpatient setting
8. What are the care processes for the patients?
  a. Deployment flowcharts
  b. Macro flowchart
9. Who cares for the patients?
  a. Interviews with staff and providers
  b. Numbers of staff
  c. Staffing schedule and patterns
10. What do patients and families say about themselves and their care?
  a. Include interviews with patients and family members
11. What are the current concerns about the care for this population of patients?
  a. Consider both a provider and patient/family perspective
12. What are the interactions of the clinical microsystem with other microsystems, the organization, and the community?
	Apply knowledge and skills to learning about illness burden of individuals in populations (MK, PC, PBLI, SBP)
	Conduct program and needs assessment and prioritize activities using objective measurable criteria, including epidemiologic impact and cost-effectiveness (SBP)
	Identify the ABNA using available metrics and standard of care (PC, MK, PBLI, SBP)
	Describe/model a clinical microsystem (SBP)
	Describe current processes of care (PC, SBP)
	Map the current process of care identify constraints to flow (SBP)
	Describe/model interactions of clinical microsystem with other microsystems, organizational context (meso- and macrosystem), and community (SBP, ICS, PC)
		When you go to the location of the care for this (these patients) patient, whom do you encounter? Who is actually involved in the care?
		How did you learn about the patients and providers?
		What surprised you as you learned about these patients and providers?
		What other information do you need?
		What did you notice that you didn't when you worked as a clinician in the microsystem?

Preliminary Development of an Aim Statement		

13. Write an initial/preliminary practicum aim.
  a. What patient population and microsystem(s) are you interested in?
  b. What care processes could be improved?
  c. What would ideal care look like for a patient in your described patient population?
  d. What are the ideal outcomes for your patient population?
		Does this work interest others at the front line?
		Is this a "reach" or realistic aim?

Resident Work and Questions for Consideration	Goals and Objectives (ACGME Core Competencies in Capital Letters)[6]	Questions Faculty Might Ask
Local Context: Local Care Problem, Care Gap		

14. Define the local care problem or care gap.
 a. What is the nature and severity of the specific local problem or system dysfunction?
 b. How do the observed processes of care lead to the results observed?
 c. Where are the constraints to care or lack of reliability?
 d. What are the impacts on patients, providers, and the institution?
   i. Patient outcomes – health, functional, satisfaction
   ii. Financial impacts – value, waste
   iii. Resources, efficiency
   iv. Use of value compass, balanced scorecard
 e. What measures are available to assess the problem?
   i. Currently abstracted and followed by microsystem and/or institution
   ii. Need to be developed by the resident and improvement team
	Describe gaps between current care and evidence (MK, PBLI, ICS, PC)
	Synthesize and present scientific evidence and its relevance to microsystem (MK, ICS, SBP, PBLI)
	Evaluate the effectiveness, accessibility, and quality of individual and population-based health-care services (PC)
	Use computers for reference retrieval, statistical analysis, graphic display, database management, and communications (PBLI)
		What is the best way to get information about the local patterns of care?
		What have you observed in the current care processes?
		What is the local perception of the problem?

Aim Statement		
15. Write global and specific aim statements a. What will be the changes/improvements in care processes and patient outcomes?	Develop and state an aim (PBLI)	Is the aim statement concise and clear?
Improvement Team		

16. Develop an improvement team.
 a. Who will be assisting you in the improvement journey? How will you connect with these people?
 b. "Microsystem mentor"
 c. Frontline staff, providers, support staff
   i. Nursing
   ii. Pharmacy
   iii. Physicians
 d. Local administrators
   i. Practice managers
   ii. Section chiefs
   iii. Medical directors
   iv. Nursing directors, leaders
 e. Senior level administrators
   i. Vice presidents
   ii. Quality and patient safety
	Synthesize and present scientific evidence and its relevance to microsystem (MK, ICS, SBP, PBLI)
	Present and share results with microsystem (ICS, SBP)
	Work effectively as a member or leader of a health-care team (SBP, P, ICS)
	Work in interprofessional teams to enhance patient safety and improve patient care quality (SBP)
		Who else needs to be on the team?
		What are the specific plans for getting the team together with regularity?

(continued)

Resident Work and Questions for Consideration	Goals and Objectives (ACGME Core Competencies in Capital Letters)[6]	Questions Faculty Might Ask
Measures		

17. Identify and define measures that can be used to assess the quality of care, based on your knowledge of the current evidence, local context, and patient population.
 	
a. How might you refine previously identified measures through a value compass or balanced scorecard approach?
  i. Narrowing down of measures that can be routinely measured
b. What are your process and outcome measures?
  i. Specific definitions of numerators and denominators for each measure
c. Where will the data be obtained and abstracted?
d. Who will perform the data collection?
e. Who will validate the data collection?
f. What is the best possible outcome for the measures?
  i. 100% – all patients should receive the care process
  ii. <100% – must be adapted to individual patient's condition or situation specific
  iii. Consideration of composite/all-or-none measures for multiple process measures
	Use value compass thinking to develop balanced measures (PBLI, MK, PC)
	Operationally define balanced measures and means for data collection/validation (PBLI)
	Prepare "dummy" and "real" data displays (ICS, PBLI)
	Using value compass thinking, develop balanced measures, methods for data collection, and means of assessing key outcomes (MK, PC, PBLI)
	Use computers for reference retrieval, statistical analysis, graphic display, database management, and communications (PBLI)
		From your review of the relevant peer-reviewed literature, what measures and levels of performance seem to be the best?
		As you begin to think about the measures you will use, what are the operational definitions of the measures and how will accurate data be gathered?
		What is the theoretical limit for this care, process, outcome?

Intervention		

18. Begin to define intervention(s) that could improve care for your patient population, based on your knowledge of the current evidence, local context, care processes, and patient population.
 	
a. Why do you think this intervention will improve care?
  i. Has this been used in other organizations successfully (benchmarking)?
  ii. Have similar interventions been reported in the literature?
b. What is your role in the implementation of the planned intervention?
  i. Leader of the improvement team or member of an existing improvement team
	Ascertain stakeholders and understand priorities (SBP, ICS, P)
	Identify organizational decision-making structures, styles, and processes (SBP)
	Identify points of leverage for change and improvement (SBP, PBLI)
	Ascertain resources available to the microsystem (individual, organizational, community) (ICS, PBLI)
	Describe/model interactions of clinical microsystem with other microsystems, organizational context, and community (SBP, ICS, PC)
		What is the underlying theory of why the proposed intervention will improve care?
		What resources or individuals should be connected?
		What are the assumptions underlying the choice of intervention?

Resident Work and Questions for Consideration	Goals and Objectives (ACGME Core Competencies in Capital Letters)[6]	Questions Faculty Might Ask
Intervention (*cont.*)		

c. What will you need to implement the planned intervention?
  i. Resources – financial, personnel, administrative
  ii. Change in practice by providers – education
  iii. Policy changes
  iv. EHR changes
d. What is the organizational decision-making process and culture in your clinical microsystem?
  i. Top-down versus consensus building
  ii. Physical artifacts, espoused beliefs and values, basic underlying assumptions
  iii. How does change occur in the microsystem?
  iv. Who are the key decision makers or influential members of the group?
  v. What is the history of improvement in the clinical microsystem? (What is the microsystem's experience with improvement? Has the microsystem tried to attempt a similar improvement intervention in the past?)
e. What are the potential challenges or barriers to successful implementation?
  i. Other competing local, regional and national priorities
  ii. Is this important to the microsystem?
f. What will your first small test of change look like?
  i. When and how will you start?
  ii. How will you study those results and proceed?
	Develop change ideas and test interventions for improvement of care (PBLI, SBP)
	Work effectively within multidisciplinary teams (SBP, P, ICS)
	Prepare and follow a realistic timeline (P, PBLI)
	Identify and describe anticipated barriers and ways to deal with them (SBP, PBLI, P)
	Identify relevant organizational and decision-making processes (P, SBP, ICS)
	Improve leadership skills (P, PBLI)
	Coordinate patient care within the health-care system (SBP)
	Develop and implement a plan to address a specific health problem (SBP)
	Manage the human and financial resources for the operation of a program or project (SBP)
		What unintended effects could occur as a result of implementing the intervention?

Ethical Issues		
19. Consider ethical aspects of implementing and studying the improvement. a. What are the privacy concerns? b. How are patients protected? c. What are the potential conflicts of interest? d. What are the potential unintended consequences of the proposed intervention?	Understand potential ethical implications of a project, and to think through appropriate responses Prepare CPHS proposal as needed Describe HIPAA implications of project Respect for patient privacy and autonomy (P)	How will you check with the appropriate ethical oversight group for the relevant ethical review of your work trying to improve this care?

(*continued*)

Resident Work and Questions for Consideration	Goals and Objectives (ACGME Core Competencies in Capital Letters)[6]	Questions Faculty Might Ask
Ethical Issues (*cont.*)		
20. Describe how you will keep data with personally identifiable information confidential and how you will determine if CPHS/IRB is needed. a. Removal of patient identifiers in database b. CPHS/IRB review of data collection and database for confidentiality 21. Submit proposed intervention and analysis plan to the CPHS/IRB for ethical review and/or quality improvement exemption.		How could patients be harmed by the proposed improvement intervention?
Analysis of Data		

22. Understand the methods that will be used to measure the impact of the intervention on the patient population
a. What aspects of the study design address internal validity (integrity of the data) and external validity (generalizability)?
b. What testing of reliability and validity of measures, assessment instruments will be performed?
c. What analytic methods will be used to determine effects of time as a variable (i.e., SPC charting)?
d. How will you know that the implemented change/intervention was adopted, changed, or rejected?
  i. Describe any quantitative and qualitative methods used to assess exposure to the intervention.
  ii. Description of the reflexivity of the intervention to the context – how did the context change the intervention and how did the intervention change the context?
23. Display and analysis of measures
a. How will you feed data back to the microsystem?
b. What are your analysis methods?
c. Where will data be displayed?
	Systematically analyze practice using QI methods and implement changes with the goal of practice improvement (PBLI)
	
	Select and conduct appropriate statistical analyses (PBLI)
	
	Use computers for reference retrieval, statistical analysis, graphic display, database management, and communications (PBLI)
	
	Incorporate considerations of cost-awareness and risk-benefit analysis in patient and/or population-based care (SBP)
	
	Apply and use information management systems (SBP)
		Who might help with study design, statistical consultation, analysis?

Outcomes		
24. Explore your results a. What changes occurred in the care processes over time – process measures, observations? b. What changes occurred in the measures of patient outcomes over time – outcome measures?	Assess organizational performance against stated goals (SBP) Conduct and evaluation or quality assessment based on process and outcome measures (SBP)	Have you plotted the data on a time plot? How were the outcomes shown to the microsystem?

Resident Work and Questions for Consideration	Goals and Objectives (ACGME Core Competencies in Capital Letters)[6]	Questions Faculty Might Ask

Outcomes (*cont.*)

   c. How were value, cost, and efficiency affected? How did you measure value?

   d. Were there unintended consequences?

Interpretation of Results and Outcomes of Intervention

25. Describe the results of the implementation of the intervention.
  a. What did you find?
  b. What were the relevant elements of the setting or context that helped or hindered the improvement work?
    i. Physical resources, organizational culture, history of change efforts
    ii. Structure and patterns of care – staffing, leadership
  c. What was the actual course of the intervention?
    i. Describe the sequence of steps, events, or phases
    ii. Type and number of participants at key points
    iii. How and why did the initial plan evolve?
      1. What lessons were learned from the evolution of the improvement process?
      2. What was the effect of internal feedback from the tests of change?
      3. Why were some interventions more successful than others?
    iv. Can use a flow chart or timeline diagram
  d. What is the evidence regarding the strength of association between observed changes/improvements and intervention components/context factors?
    i. What makes you think that the interventions led to the observed improvements? Could other factors be more responsible for observed changes?
    ii. Present data on exposure to the intervention
	Develop, deliver, and implement appropriate clinical services for both individuals and populations in order to diagnose and treat medical problems and chronic conditions (PC)
	
	Participate in the education of patients, families, students, residents and other health professionals (PBLI)
	
	(Apply primary, secondary, and tertiary approaches to individual and population-based disease prevention and health promotion [PC])
	
	(Develop, implement, and evaluate the effectiveness of appropriate clinical preventive services for both individuals and populations [PC])
	
	(Implement programs to reduce the exposure to risk factors for an illness or a condition in a population [PC])
		What was the effect of the intervention on the microsystem?
		
		What was the effect of the microsystem/context on the intervention?
		
		How did the intervention change over time and why?
		
		What other local or national trends could explain the findings?
		
		Be careful to note any changes that occurred as the intervention unfolded. Be sure to keep notes in real time.
		
		As you think about the limitations, think as broadly as possible

(*continued*)

Resident Work and Questions for Consideration	Goals and Objectives (ACGME Core Competencies in Capital Letters)[6]	Questions Faculty Might Ask

Interpretation of Results and Outcomes of Intervention (*cont.*)

   f. How do your findings compare to other published studies or experiences at other similar institutions?

26. Explore the limitations of your findings.

   a. What are possible sources of confounding, bias, or imprecision in design, measurement, and analysis that may have affected study outcomes (internal validity)?

   b. What factors could affect generalizability (external validity)?

   i.   Representativeness of participants

   ii. Effectiveness of implementation

   iii. Dose-response effects

   iv. Features of local context, setting

Reflections and Next Steps

27. Reflect on successes and difficulties in implementing the improvement interventions

   a. What were the main changes observed in care delivery and clinical outcomes?

   b. How do these compare with what you expected?

   c. What are the factors that produced these results?

28. Plan for sustainability

   a. What is the likelihood that the observed improvements will continue over time?

   b. What are the plans for continued monitoring of measures and care processes and maintaining improvements?

   c. Who is involved with the transition plan?

   d. What can be done to improve future performance over time?

29. Lessons learned

   a. What would you have done differently?

   b. What was successful and why?

   c. What is the future of the intervention?

   d. What are the implications of the improvement work?

   i.   Planned improvement work

   ii. Change in context, culture, beliefs in the local setting

   e. What are the implications for your future work and professional development?

   f. What advice would you give to others?

Work effectively as a member or leader of a health-care team to enhance patient safety and improve patient care quality (ICS, P, SBP)

Identify organizational decision-making structures, stakeholders, styles, and processes (SBP)

Demonstrate skills in management and administration (SBP)

Assess organizational performance against stated goals (SBP)

Identify strengths, deficiencies, and limits in one's knowledge and expertise (PBLI)

How were you changed by this work?

What would you not do again?

What advice would you give to others who follow you?

How will your practice change?

What have you learned about leadership and change in a health care setting?

How has the microsystem changed because of your efforts?

Resident Work and Questions for Consideration	Goals and Objectives (ACGME Core Competencies in Capital Letters)[6]	Questions Faculty Might Ask
Dissemination of Results		
30. Share your experiences and findings with others. a. What are your plans for publication? Who will coauthor your manuscript? b. What are your plans for local and nonlocal presentation?	Use computers for reference retrieval, statistical analysis, graphic display, database management, and communications (PBLI) Advocate for quality patient care and optimal patient care systems (SBP) Communicate effectively with physicians, other health professionals, and health related agencies (ICS)	What is your timeline? What are the best venues for sharing this information (both internal and external)? How might you approach different audiences?

Abbreviations: ACGME, Accreditation Council on Graduate Medical Education; ABNA, achievable benefit not achieved; CMS, Centers for Medicare and Medicaid Services; CPHS, Committee for the Protection of Human Subjects; ED, emergency department; EHR, electronic health record; HIPAA, Health Insurance Portability and Accountability Act; ICS, interpersonal and communication skills; IRB, Institutional Review Board; JCAHO, Joint Commission on Accreditation of Healthcare Organizations; LOS, length of stay; MK, medical knowledge; NQF, National Quality Forum; P, professionalism; PBLI, practice-based learning and improvement; PC, patient care; QI, quality improvement; SBP, systems-based practice; SPC, statistical process control.

What Are Our Outcomes?
• •

Residents have worked on a wide variety of topics, as shown in Table 5.2.

TABLE 5.2 Program Combinations and Practicum Work

Specialty Program Combinations: Preventive Medicine and ...	Practicum Focus
Internal medicine	Inpatient care for community-acquired pneumonia
Family practice	Improving obesity care at a family health center
Internal medicine	Coordination of care for newly diagnosed pancreatic cancer
Family practice	Pediatric immunizations
Anesthesiology	Sedation outside the operating room
Gastroenterology	Colonoscopy withdrawal times
Pain medicine	Use of epidurals for post-op pain control
Family practice	Teen clinic at a rural family health center
Family practice	Care plans for complex patients
Internal medicine	Outpatient diabetes care
Infectious disease	Hand hygiene in same-day surgery
Internal medicine	Inpatient diabetes care
Infectious disease	Preparing patients for home intravenous antibiotic therapy
Pathology	Platelet supply in the blood bank
Psychiatry	Depression care in resident psychopharmacology clinic
Endocrinology	Screening for diabetes in general internal medicine
Surgery	Deep vein thrombosis prophylaxis in surgery
Surgery	Advance directives for head and neck cancer patients
Surgery	Improving trauma team readiness
Obstetrics-gynecology	HIV screening in pregnancy
Pediatrics	Improving pediatric obesity care
Critical care	Rapid response team implementation
Infectious disease	Improving time to first dose of antibiotics
Neonatology	Decreasing ventilator days in the intensive care nursery
Obstetrics-gynecology	Postoperative complications in urogynecology
Family practice	Advance directives for frail elderly in the family health center
Pathology	Decreasing specimen labeling errors
Family practice	Shared medical appointments for diabetes

Not all practicums result in sustained improvement, but many do. Habits of work and conversation have changed, and workgroups continue to meet and improve care even after the involved resident has graduated. Many have produced significant system changes, such as the creation of a sedation service, revamping of the acute pain service, creation of a microsystem focused on pediatric obesity, new models of care such as shared medical appointments, new care plan templates in a system-wide electronic health record, and tools to improve discussion and documentation of advance directives in an entire community. A number of publications have come from our residents' work and they continue to share their results broadly.[5,8–12]

Graduates of the program have gone on to a variety of work settings. Some return to their "home" programs to finish training or pursue fellowships. The vast majority who have transitioned out of training programs are in positions in which they explicitly play a role in system improvement, in both academic and nonacademic settings. Some are working in more "traditional" public health settings such as the US Centers for Disease Control, but all are employed in jobs of choice.

What Have We Learned?

Over time, we have seen that every resident's journey through the program is unique, responding to different clinical settings where the work takes place, different coach/resident "chemistry," and different challenges and opportunities. However, looking back over our first 8 years of experience, we also saw that the resident journeys touched on a set of similar questions, captured in the developmental journey described. Intending originally to flesh out the details of the rough framework which we had provided in a set of goals and expectations, we found that we had created a document that called out the triangle in a series of questions – questions that can only be answered with deep knowledge of the patients and their outcomes, the factors that create the care system's performance, and an understanding of who is involved. Answering these questions and working with everyone involved in care results in professional development for not only resident and coach, but also their team members and others affected by the improvement work.

We have learned much about helping residents and fellows develop skills in leading change and improving care. We have also learned a tremendous amount about the medical centers where we work and our connections to the community borne of the residents' public health work. We have learned an enormous amount about ourselves, as faculty, administrators, and adult learners. We have learned about what it takes to make the triangle real – moving out from our corner of professional development into the world of outcomes and systems, and what it takes to invite and involve everyone in that work. We have learned about how to describe the work we are doing, though we continue to refine those descriptions. We have learned that the triangle is an important orienting image for those descriptions. Most important, we have learned that the triangle is real – inhabited by real patients, encompassing real systems populated by real people who want to provide the best care possible for those patients, and who bring great creativity and dedication to that work, pushing the boundaries and growing their own skills and reflective capacity as they care for others, and each other. We have learned what it takes to support and help each other. We have learned to be grateful for these opportunities, and for the hard work of all involved.

References

1. Ducatman AM, Vanderploeg JM, Johnson M, *et al*. Residency training in preventive medicine: challenges and opportunities. *Am J Prev Med*. 2005; **28**(4): 403–12.
2. Program Management Group, DHLPMR Program Policies and Procedures (unpublished).
3. Cooperrider DL, Sorenson PF, Whitney D, *et al*. *Appreciative Inquiry: rethinking human organization toward a positive theory of change*. Champaign, IL: Stipes Publishing; 1999.
4. Glouberman S, Zimmerman B. *Complicated and Complex Systems: what would successful reform of Medicare look like?* Discussion Paper No. 8. Commission on the Future of Health Care in Canada; July, 2002.
5. Liu SK, Homa K, Butterly JR, *et al*. Improving the simple, complicated and complex realities of community-acquired pneumonia. *Qual Saf Health Care*. 2009; **18**(2): 93–8.
6. www.squire-statement.org
7. www.acgme.org
8. Shiner B, Green RL, Homa K, *et al*. Improving depression care in a psychiatry resident psychopharmacology clinic: measurement, monitoring, feedback, and education. *Qual Saf Health Care*. 2010; **19**(3): 234–8.
9. Pastel LC, Liu S, Homa K, *et al*. Improving care for patients with diabetes at a rural primary care clinic by empowering licensed nursing assistants with a flow sheet tool. *Clin Diabetes*. 2009; **27**(3): 115–18.
10. Prairie BA, Foster T. Improving prenatal HIV screening with tailored educational interventions: an approach to guideline implementation. *Qual Saf Health Care*. 2010; **19**(6): 1–5.
11. Chen JJ, Conway M, Kanakis A, *et al*. Do hospital-based delirium prevention programs work? A systematic review and meta-analysis. *J Am Geriatrics Soc*. 2010; **58**(S1): 219.
12. Trummel JT, Surgenor S, Cravero JP, *et al*. Comparison of differing sedation practice for upper endoscopic ultrasound using expert observational analysis of the procedural sedation. *J Patient Saf*. 2009; **5**(3): 153–9.

6

Simple, Complicated, and Complex Phenomena in Health Care

Using the Triangle to Improve Reliability *and* Resiliency in Health-Care Systems

Stephen Liu, Tina Foster, and Paul Batalden

It's the morning of "go-live," the first day of implementation of a new electronic health record (EHR) with computerized provider order entry (CPOE) and it seems like every aspect of how I practice medicine has been changed.

I've just started morning rounds and the first patient I see is a 64-year-old gentleman with a history of obesity and cardiac disease who was transferred overnight from a local community hospital for worsening renal failure. Shortly after I leave his room, he calls out that he is experiencing left-sided chest pain that is radiating to his jaw and down his left arm. After examining the patient, I quickly decide that he needs an EKG and labs/cardiac enzymes drawn as soon as possible. I type "EKG" into the order entry field in the new EHR and fill out the five required fields to complete the order. After spending several minutes ensuring that the required fields are complete I ask the nurse whether she received the order. She turns to her own computer but can't locate the order for the EKG. We reach out to the local nursing and physician EHR content experts that were on the floor to help out with the implementation; it takes some time, but, they are finally able to locate the order for the EKG. However, the assembled group is now unsure whether the electronic order has actually notified the EKG technician to come to the unit to perform the EKG. Additionally, the nurses are not sure where the labels have printed out for the blood draws and are not sure whether the phlebotomist is aware of the need for an urgent blood draw. Finally, we give up on using the computer system and page the EKG technician and phlebotomist over the phone. The EKG technician and phlebotomist arrive promptly, but now need a "requisition" through the computer to complete the orders. The enlarging group of health-care providers huddle around one computer to try and figure out what needs to be done to provide appropriate care for a patient who needs urgent attention.

At this point it has taken well over 30 minutes and everyone is increasingly frustrated and angry at the new EHR and those who have spent the last 4 years working on implementation. We wonder why we spent hours in a classroom practicing in the "playground" but never had the opportunity to test questions such as these. The ordering of STAT labs was yet another area that had not been fleshed out and practiced prior to go-live. Two days ago, we used to be able to do this easily, everyone knew how to obtain an EKG and blood draws. It used to be so simple: I just wrote "EKG and cardiac enzymes ×3" on a paper order sheet and signed my name. Now I've been stuck in front of a computer for the past 30 minutes with a group of six other health-care providers trying to figure out how to provide proper and timely care for a patient. Why are we doing this? This EHR has been implemented successfully in dozens of other hospitals in the country, so why is our hospital having such a hard time? Things worked fine before, now this new system is changing everything. It's wasting everyone's time! This change is hurting patients!

Transforming health care to improve quality is not for the faint of heart. To improve all three elements of the triangle (patient and population outcomes, system performance and professional development) simultaneously requires conceptual frameworks to help along the journey as it is not always clear what improvement interventions to consider for a particular problem or care gap that exists.

Health care and the problems it presents to anyone seeking to improve it invites understanding and study. We put names on the types of problems that we recognize as an aid in addressing them. We have found that discerning the difference between simple, complicated and complex aspects of challenges is a useful construct for practicing physicians and leaders of health-care systems in the design of improvement interventions.

Simple, Complicated, and Complex Problems in Health Care
•••••••••••••••

Glouberman and Zimmerman[1] and Zimmerman et al.[2] have suggested that there are at least three types of problems that can be recognized in health care. One type can be thought of as "simple." The elements of the system involved are known and their relationships are understood and stable. The causal system of the *simple* health-care problem is known and predictable. Zimmerman and others have used the metaphor of the challenge of making cookies where recipes can help the baker. Making the causal system explicit (often by graphic representation) can help in the effort to redesign and to make the health care involved reliable. An example of a simple scenario in the health-care system is influenza vaccinations. There is convincing scientific evidence that receiving an influenza vaccination has significant benefits that outweigh the risks to patients. In deciding who should get the vaccination, there are clear guidelines and recommendations and there is little room for physician judgment in adapting these guidelines for a particular patient. These problems invite clear standards: if something should be done, a forcing function or a checklist can help. Similarly, if something should not be done, a forcing function to prevent it can be useful. Standing orders for vaccinations, automatic stop orders for indwelling urinary catheters and certain aspects of checklists are examples of improvement interventions designed to address simple "yes" or "no" problems.

A second type of health-care problem involves contingent phenomena. They called these problems "complicated." The elements, relationships, and causal system in the *complicated* problem in health care are "knowable." Exploring and testing cause/effect relations can help redesign and make the related health care predictable and reliable. Glouberman and Zimmerman[1] use the metaphor of "sending a rocket to the moon" as an example. Multiple streams of knowledge may be involved and linked. Their interaction can be facilitated with algorithms, which specify desired action in the contingent reality of the *complicated* health care we encounter. An example of a complicated scenario is a clinical or care pathway for patients undergoing cardiac bypass surgery. Each step in the care process is laid out in detail and is contingent upon meeting certain patient parameters. The care process has been developed from the experiences of a population of similar patients and the expertise of experienced clinicians. Yet another example is a protocol to administer an intravenous insulin infusion where if a diabetic patient's blood glucose is at or above a certain level, specific instructions on adjusting the rate of infusion are detailed. Further adjustments are based upon the subsequent blood glucose readings and the next steps in adjusting the rate of the insulin are clearly defined based on known patient characteristics. Complicated problems invite an understanding of the contingent ("if, then") realities encountered in health care.

The third type of problem Glouberman and Zimmerman[1] name as "complex." They describe it as involving elements and relationships that can change, making reliability elusive. The causal system of *complex* phenomena is not stable, and therefore unknowable. They use the metaphor of raising children – success with the first child in a family does not predict success with the second. While some advice or guidelines are helpful, the ultimate outcome is not always predictable because of the number of different variables that can affect the outcome. Because the causal system is unstable and cannot be known, these health-care phenomena can aim to become more or less resilient, if not reliable. Attention to the aim and relationships of the people in the complex situation can help. For example, the care of a patient with multiple chronic medical conditions, such as diabetes, heart disease, and obesity, with an unstable home situation would be considered a complex problem. Although there are certainly evidence based guidelines or treatment recommendations for each of the chronic medical conditions, in a single patient these guidelines may contradict one another or they may not be appropriate given the patient's personal treatment goals. While a particular treatment may make sense in a large population of patients, it must be considered in the specific context of the patient's other health conditions and their values, wishes, and goals in care. Complex problems invite attention to the relationships and the shared aim of those involved. These situations require significant provider judgment and autonomy to tailor the care for a particular patient and context (*see* Table 6.1).

TABLE 6.1 A Description of Simple, Complicated, and Complex Problems as They Relate to Health-Care Improvement

	Simple Problems, "All or None"	Complicated Problems, "If/Then"	Complex Problems, "Relational/Maybe"
Typical Health-Care Process or Problem	• Obtaining vital signs and assessment of oxygenation status • Assessing vaccination history and providing vaccinations as indicated • Administering prophylactic antibiotics in the preoperative period • Washing hands prior to patient contact	• Intravenous insulin titration for a patient with diabetic ketoacidosis • Care pathways designed for patients undergoing cardiac bypass surgery	• Adapting treatment plans to reflect patient and family wishes in end-of-life care • Management of multiple chronic medical conditions in a homeless patient without health insurance • Improving readmissions in patients with multiple medical conditions

	Simple Problems, "All or None"	Complicated Problems, "If/Then"	Complex Problems, "Relational/Maybe"
Implementation of Recommended Care Process and Patient Autonomy/Input into Care Plan	• Every patient should or should not receive care process • Typically, benefits outweigh risks so specific patient and provider decision making/input is low	• Conditions of preferred use are known/discoverable but need to be adapted to specific patient input/values	• Patient and family input/ values and influence of co-occurring medical conditions significantly determine treatment plan
Expected Outcome	• Known • Predictable based on outcome results from studies and previous experiences	• Knowable • Largely predictable based on previous experiences with similar patients	• Partly known • Essentially unpredictable because of the unique combination of patient characteristics and clinical uncertainty about treatments
Scientific Evidence/ Literature about Treatment Options	• Broad scientific agreement that the treatments/processes improve outcome measures (morbidity and mortality)	• Patients who receive care that is appropriate for their clinical condition have improved outcomes	• Treatment guidelines and evidence may not be applicable to a specific patient due to patient's preferences and characteristics • Treatment guidelines may conflict in patients with multiple co-occurring conditions
Ideal Level of Provider Autonomy	Low	Variable	High
Potential Improvement Interventions	• Certain aspects of checklists • Standing orders for vaccinations • Forcing functions	• Standard admission orders • Care pathways • Standardized protocols and guidelines for patient conditions	• Provide space and time to encourage development of relationships between providers and patients/ families
Oversight/ Monitoring	• Public reporting of quality measures	• Feedback to providers • Public reporting of quality measures	• Look for patterns of interventions and outcomes • Examine disease burden of patient and families • Provider and patient/ family satisfaction with care
Improvement Aim	Increased reliability	Increased reliability	Increased resiliency

Matching Problem Type with Improvement Interventions

Understanding the type of problem or clinical scenario at hand can help improve the design of associated improvement interventions. Properly matching an intervention to the real situation has the potential to greatly increase the success and uptake among the health-care team. For example, if one were trying to increase vaccination rates among patients being discharged from a hospital (a simple "yes/no" scenario), one could consider a "forcing function" intervention where patients cannot be discharged unless their vaccination status is assessed and they are vaccinated as appropriate prior to discharge (a simple intervention). However, if one is trying to improve a complex system (i.e., a health-care institution with multiple inpatient units and outpatient clinics) or complex problem (i.e., end-of-life care, hospital readmissions), a complex multifaceted intervention is likely required in order to make meaningful change and work on the establishment of a shared aim and interdependent relationships is likely a good place to begin.

Frequently, the argument is made that improvement interventions such as checklists or standardized care pathways are not flexible enough to adjust for the individual variation needed to optimize patient care. The logical extension of this argument is that providers should not be constrained in the care that they provide to patients. The simple, complicated, and complex framework allows one to accommodate both points of view in the design of health-care systems and improvement interventions. The goal of well-designed systems should be increased reliability through increased standardization (with attention to the underlying science and appropriate constraints on provider autonomy) in simple and complicated scenarios and increased provider autonomy and judgment (with fewer constraints in care through standardization) in complex situations or problems.

To increase value, the aim should be to increase standardization in simple and complicated scenarios or problems, and at the same time seek to increase provider autonomy, judgment, and flexibility in complex scenarios where the aim is increased resiliency. This distinction allows providers to use their skills and talents to tailor care for complex situations while at the same time taking "simpler" aspects of care away from the provider by standardizing care that does not need specific input from providers.

> Later on that afternoon, the patient's chest pain had resolved and he had received the necessary EKG and lab work that did not show any evidence of a cardiac cause for the chest pain. With space and time to reflect during the afternoon, I began to examine some of the changes that were occurring with implementation of this new computer system and thought about aspects of our "old" paper-based system that had been in place just the day before.

Taking care of patients before the implementation of the EHR used to be so "simple." We had three paper binders that were located in three different locations near a patient's room. One green binder contained the papers to write orders, and it had paper copies of EKG's and nursing notes; the second, pink binder contained vital signs, input/output data, and nursing care notes; a third, tan-colored binder had a handwritten list of all the medications that were given to a patient with times that they were given or held.

Unfortunately, this "simple" noncomputerized system also had many downsides. One often had to search around the nursing area for these binders, as they were frequently misplaced or left in a patient's room. One of the most common sources of medication errors that occurred in this system was transcription errors. Messy handwriting for orders could be misinterpreted by a nurse who was reading a physician's order. Illegible signatures made it impossible to determine who wrote orders. Nurses who copied orders could make mistakes and change doses or frequencies of intended medications.

In selected patient populations, electronic health records with computerized provider order entry have been shown to improve patient outcomes and system performance. EHRs can also help with professional development by incorporating education into patient care orders and the inclusion of evidence-based order sets to help improve the medical knowledge of providers. A new EHR eliminates the need for paper documentation and keeps all the required patient data in a single location. EHRs also have the ability to include safety checks for medications – checking allergies, drug interactions, and alerting providers of best practices based on a patient's medications and diagnoses. Use of CPOE with clinical decision support systems has been shown to reduce medical errors and adverse drug events, improve health outcomes, reduce health-care costs, and improve management of certain chronic conditions.[3–7]

Based on this evidence and other economic and financial incentives, increasing numbers of hospitals and health-care institutions are adopting EHRs and CPOE. At the same time, implementation of these complicated computerized systems can be fraught with difficulties. Adoption of a new EHR touches on all aspects of medical care throughout a health-care institution and there are thousands of contingencies that need to be considered and prepared for prior to implementation.

Care processes, staff responsibilities, and patient flow must all be carefully mapped out so that an EHR can support staff in their efforts to provide the best care for each patient. With a lot of planning and work, most institutions have successfully implemented EHRs. Given the complex nature of health care, these discussions require substantial understanding of how the work is actually done and negotiating agreement about the key steps and their ownership. Granted, some institutions have had great technical difficulties with implementation but most of these glitches are usually solvable with the right technical expertise. However, the context of implementation requires consideration, given that most clinical microsystems where the EHR will be used are complex adaptive systems.

Health-Care Systems as Complex Adaptive Systems

Health-care systems, whether they are small primary care clinics with one physician provider or 50-bed inpatient units with dozens of different physician and nursing providers, can all be considered components of complex adaptive systems. Patients seen in a primary care clinic can be hospitalized in an acute care facility, referred to specialist providers, undergo surgeries in tertiary care facilities, and can be admitted to local nursing homes or rehabilitation facilities. The interactions and the resulting relationships that develop between patients and providers of the various microsystems within a given health-care system are all components of complex adaptive systems. Melanie Mitchell,[8] in *Complexity: A Guided Tour*, has described the following common properties of complex adaptive systems.

- *Complex collective behavior*: complex adaptive systems consist of large networks of individual components with each following simple rules. The collective actions of the individual components lead to the observed patterns of behavior. In a large health-care institution with multiple inpatient units and outpatient clinics, each of the respective units or clinics interacts with one another yet each is also governed by a set of rules, norms, and culture that is specific to the individual unit.

- *Signaling and information processing*: complex systems "produce and use information and signals from both their internal and external environments." In a health-care system, these signals take the form of medical records (whether they are electronic or paper based), telephone communication, or patient communication and reports of findings between different providers and institutions.

- *Adaptation*: each of the components of the complex system have the ability to adapt or evolve over time. In health care, while some aspects of care are similar from year to year, each individual clinic or provider is constantly responding to numerous external and internal changes (financial reimbursement, institutional policy changes, regulatory changes) over time. Some of these changes may be minor but others may be much more dramatic, such as the implementation of a new electronic health record.

Mitchell has further defined a complex adaptive system as "a system in which large networks of components with no central control and simple rules of operation give rise to complex collective behavior, sophisticated information processing, and adaptation via learning or evolution."[8] This definition would certainly be applicable to most health-care systems with multiple units, clinics, or providers.

> Two weeks after the launch of the EHR, many physicians are still upset about the fact that they cannot provide care in the manner they want to … or at least used to. They feel that the adoption of the EHR is interfering with their work and their ability to provide optimal patient care. By the same token, there are also many who have embraced the new technology and see how the new systems of care are improving patient care. Each individual and section adapted to the implementation of the new EHR in a slightly different way. Some sections held multiple training sessions and "dress rehearsals" many months prior to implementation, while others had minimal amounts of training and preparation. As a result, some individuals and clinics within the institution adapted well to the change, whereas others struggled with the change.

The adoption of a new EHR is not a complicated problem – it is complex. While the mechanics of installing a new computer system could be considered complicated, a new EHR perturbs the traditions in the way physicians and other care providers go about their work making it a complex problem. It challenges the culture, the norms, the traditions, and the relationships in the system. On the surface, the only apparent change is writing orders through a computer rather than in a paper chart. However, the ways in which these orders are communicated have also changed. Previously, a provider would come to a patient's room, write an order in the paper chart, and discuss the new order with the patient's nurse and the patient. With the advent of CPOE, orders could now be written anywhere in and outside the hospital and nurses were notified of new orders when they log into a patient's chart electronically. As a result, the communication and relationship patterns between nurse and physician and physician and patient had been drastically altered with the advent of new technology.

Like raising a child, certain advice and guidelines are helpful but each individual's experience is slightly different and unpredictable in terms of the end-result and outcome. Simple and complicated problems lend themselves to one answer with an outcome that is largely predictable. There is usually one correct way to address the problem. But complex challenges have many right answers that could lead to a desired outcome. There is no one right way that will work for all. Instead, there are multiple good ways – as there are in child rearing. It is context dependent and deals with emergent unpredictable elements. This is the reason why implementing a new EHR and CPOE is not the same in different institutions. Each particular context must adapt the use of the EHR to the particular setting, practices, and culture. Computerized health records are a proposed solution to help improve the quality, safety, and efficiency of a health-care system. The implementation of an EHR is in essence a complex challenge with some simple and complicated elements. The huge number of interdependencies, relationships, connections, and unpredictable reactions created an overall complex problem.

Reliability versus Resilience

It's been 1 month since "go-live" and things have been chaotic throughout the hospital. Many providers have had significant difficulties in integrating the new EHR into their work flows and care processes. As a result, there continue to be major inefficiencies and many providers are spending significantly more time caring for the same number of patients. Additionally, care processes that used to ensure follow-up are not supported in the new EHR (or do not seem adequately reliable to the providers). As a result, many providers developed "work-arounds" to ensure that patients continued to receive the best care possible. These "work-arounds" included writing down pending lab tests on pieces of paper, calling in prescriptions, and e-mailing notes rather than relying on the EHR to take care of those tasks.

In a complex health-care system, staff and providers quickly adapt to new changes and develop novel techniques to ensure that their patients receive proper care. These so-called "work-arounds" can identify areas in which the system is not performing well and also identify areas in which improvement work can be directed.

Although implementing an EHR was a significant institutional change that affected every health-care provider, the essential aspects of providing health care were largely unchanged, particularly from the patient's perspective. Nurses, physicians, and others still developed relationships with patients; patients and families were still involved in shared decision making with providers; and needed medical interventions and procedures still occurred. Granted, for some providers it took much longer to provide the care with the new system and it was perceived to be less efficient. However, all providers eventually adapted to ensure that all their patients received the best care possible. Even though previous ways of accomplishing tasks were not available, there were other pathways to provide the care that was needed.

Looking through the lens of a complex adaptive system, a "simple rule" of health-care systems is that providers will do whatever it takes to ensure that patients receive the best care possible. As can be seen in the example of an EHR implementation, providers will quickly adapt and evolve to ensure that this simple rule is followed. Encouraging provider autonomy and flexibility in adapting work processes to follow simple rules of patient care can help improve outcomes and at times, system performance. For complex systems or problems, one size does not fit all and each intervention must consider the particular context prior to implementation to ensure success. Encouraging provider autonomy in designing individual workflow solutions ensures resiliency to optimize patient outcomes. It needs to be emphasized that the improvement aim for *simple and complicated* problems is increased reliability with decreased variability in care processes. One would seek to reduce unnecessary variations in aspects of simple or complicated care and eliminate "work-arounds" while allowing greater provider flexibility in addressing complex problems. This highlights the importance of identifying the problem that exists and matching the improvement intervention or strategy accordingly.

Expect Unintended Consequences

One particularly troubling aspect of the new EHR to the outpatient pediatric clinics was the requirement to verify a patient's weight in the system before entering an order. The intent of the requirement was to ensure that the weight-based dosing often used in pediatrics would be correct. However, it was discovered after "go-live" that some pediatric patients had multiple appointments on the same day, which required multiple weight verifications. This meant that some patients had to be weighed several times in the same day. This extra step was thought to be time-consuming and inefficient. As a result, it was decided to remove this requirement from the system.

Unfortunately, changes made in the outpatient pediatric clinic also affected the entire system including the inpatient setting and adult patients. At the time of the decision, it was thought that there would not be negative consequences for adult inpatients because a pharmacist reviews and verifies all medication doses before they are dispensed. However, after the weight requirement was removed, several hospitalized pediatric and adult patients received the wrong dose of a medication. In the analysis of the medication errors, it was found that for patients who did not have a weight entered into the system, the first dose could be "auto-verified" in certain units and thus bypassed pharmacist review and allowed errors to reach a patient.

One of the principal characteristics of complex systems is emergence. Novel events can emerge that would not be anticipated based on what could have been predicted based on the knowledge of the individual elements within a system. In this particular case, a change made to accommodate the pediatric clinics affected the care for hospitalized adults. Owing to the interconnectedness of complex health-care systems, changes made in one setting can have significant impacts in non-related settings that cannot always be predicted beforehand. Given this characteristic, one needs to be prepared for these to occur by actively monitoring for both known and unknown effects of system changes in complex systems.

Unintended effects of interventions are not always detrimental and can often be helpful and produce desired outcomes. Some minor changes that occur in a clinic or inpatient unit can have dramatic results to the larger institution or community at large. One particular instance of this occurred with a group attempting to improve care for hospitalized pneumonia patients. This improvement effort engaged an initially small group of individuals that designed some discharge interventions to ensure that patients who were active tobacco users were referred to a telephone quit line and prescribed nicotine replacement therapy at the time of discharge to home. While this improvement group initially focused on the care for a population of pneumonia patients, the positive work of this group and the identification of a lack of resources for tobacco users in the institution and the community led to the creation of a dedicated Tobacco Treatment Team. This team spearheaded the spread of the telephone quit line referral process to all other inpatient units, created an outpatient tobacco cessation class and an inpatient cessation consult service. Additionally, the efforts of the Tobacco Treatment Team contributed to the implementation of a smoke-free campus at the hospital and led to a ban on cigarette sales at a local grocery store.[9] These significant and sustained changes in a health-care setting and the surrounding community were started with an initial improvement project in a single inpatient unit in a hospital. This example highlights the power of emergence in improvement work and the unpredictable ways in which the hard work and enthusiasm of a small group can develop into a larger movement that could not have been predicted at the outset.

Complexity and the Triangle

Improvement interventions that are matched to the clinical scenario or problem that exists allows for the greatest chances of success and sustainability for the improvement work. Unfortunately, mismatches in improvement work are far too common where the proposed improvement intervention does not match the problem that exists. Mismatched improvement interventions can lead to frustrated providers who know that the extra work involved with a particular intervention is unlikely to improve the problem it was designed to address.

Over the past several years, significant resources have been devoted to improving readmission rates throughout the country. Readmissions could certainly be considered a complex problem occurring among patients with multiple chronic medical conditions who receive care in a complex health-care system involving inpatient and outpatient care settings. Unfortunately, interventions that only address simple or complicated aspects of a complex problem and are unlikely to result in lasting improvements to patient care are implemented. For instance, many institutions have implemented discrete interventions to improve readmissions such as follow-up phone calls or scheduling follow-up visits after discharge. A recent meta-analysis that evaluated over 300 published studies on readmission improvement work found that no single intervention was associated with a reduced risk of 30-day readmission rates.[10] Patients return to a hospital and need to be readmitted for a vast array of reasons that are dependent upon their health and functional status and the social and family support in their home environment. Delving deeper into the literature, multifaceted improvement interventions that involved "transition coaches" along with bundles of improvement interventions such as patient-centered discharge instructions and improvements in outpatient care have had success in improving rates of readmissions. It is likely that these complex multifaceted interventions promoted the development of significant provider-patient relationships and shared aims that were ultimately responsible for the observed improvements in readmissions and overall patient care.

This does not mean that simple or complicated interventions should not be attempted for complex problems. It is the process of improving the care for a population of patients that often leads to complex changes within a given system. The creation of an improvement team that engages providers and patients in the improvement process to implement a seemingly "simple" change can often have dramatic changes in a particular setting by changing the culture of a given microsystem and the relationships between providers and patients within. The invitation to change something seems to "recruit" greater sharing of the common aim and the relationships that are necessary to realize that aim. So in these cases, the process of improvement with resulting changes in cultural norms can often be more important than the specifics of a given improvement intervention. Alternatively, ignoring these relationships and contextual issues and implementing a simple or complicated solution for a complex solution is unlikely to lead to meaningful, sustained improvements in health care.

The triangle allows this balanced, multifaceted approach to improving complex problems in health-care institutions. By examining systems through each lens of the triangle (patient outcomes, professional development, and system performance) one can begin to envision the interventions needed to implement real change in health-care systems. It can also help identify improvement interventions that are only directed at one aspect of the triangle, which will highlight the unintended effects on the other two points of the triangle. If one works only

TABLE 6.2 Matrix of Clarifying Questions between the Problem that Needs to be Addressed and the Aim of the Triangle

Type of Problem/ Aim	Better Outcome	Better System Performance	Better Professional Development
Simple	• Causal system explicit? • Measures of process, outcome clear, done regularly?	• Quality, safety, value clearly defined? • Measured regularly?	• "Known" process understood by professionals involved? • Role of other professionals known and understood?
Complicated	• Contingencies mapped to intended outcomes? • Measured well? • Measurement integrated with ongoing "knowledge building" of the process?	• Contingencies integrated with algorithms of care, documentation? • Impact of contingencies on quality, safety, value known, documented?	• "Knowable" process, contingencies understood by professionals involved? • Role of other professionals understood, anticipated?
Complex	• Aim clear? • Relation to desired outcomes explicit? • Patient, family share aim?	• Aim measurably defined and regularly measured? • Adaptive capacities measured, documented, improved?	• Relationships between and among professionals and between professionals and beneficiaries known, supportive of aim? • Relation of shared aim and sense of "meaning" in professional work known?

on professional development, this could come at the expense of patient outcomes or system performance.

An example of this was the change made by the Accreditation Council on Graduate Medical Education (ACGME) to regulate resident physician work hours in the United States. In 2003, the ACGME mandated that resident physicians could not work for more than 80 hours per week and should have on average 1 day off per week. While this was a needed change, it also had significant effects on system performance. The unintended side effects of this change were increases in discontinuity in patient care by increasing the numbers of hand-offs in care. In terms of system performance and value, the costs associated with increased staffing needs due to changes in resident work hours have been estimated at $1.6 billion.[11]

In this particular case, the complex problem is the challenge of providing safe and effective care for patients in an academic health sciences center while at the same time ensuring that resident physicians have a safe and protected learning environment during their training process. Using the triangle to examine this problem, one can see that restricting work hours was clearly designed to improve professional development and to some extent patient outcomes by improving patient safety; however, the effects on the performance of the system of these changes were not clearly measured or broadly anticipated prior to implementation.

By evaluating complex problems and proposed interventions through all three points of the triangle, one can be better prepared to measure the intended and unintended effects of the interventions to improve patient care.

We have found that a matrix of questions integrating simple, complicated, and complex problems with the three-part aims of better outcomes, better system performance, and better professional development of the triangle can help identify the problem that exists and identify issues that need to be addressed to improve each point of the triangle.

Conclusions

Now it is 6 months since "go-live." Things are settling down and overall, have improved. Clinicians are beginning to get a sense of how the new system might improve patient care by making it more safe and reliable. Further adjustments to improve efficiency have occurred along with educational sessions with providers. Individual providers are learning the best ways to utilize the new EHR and are teaching colleagues and residents about these "tips and tricks" to optimize the use of CPOE and the EHR. Overall, patient care has returned to previous levels of efficiency and providers are integrating the system into their daily practice. Providers are also beginning to understand the potential of the new EHR and projects to harness the data reporting capabilities and integration of evidence-based medicine and decision support into patient care are under development.

Change in the health-care system is inevitable. Changes in technology and financing will continue to shape how patients and providers interact in the future. Dealing with these changes in an increasingly complex system will become a necessary skill for future health-care providers and leaders. Clearly identifying the problem that exists in a particular context or health-care setting and then matching it to a potential solution will give an improvement intervention the best chances of initial and sustained success. Additionally, well-matched and well-designed improvement interventions are better integrated into clinical work processes and feel less like additional work that does not provide value to the patient or provider. The overall goal for improvement work should be to increase the reliability and standardization of simple and complicated problems so that providers can have increased autonomy and resilience in dealing with complex problems. This will ultimately decrease the amount of time providers spend on tasks that can be automated by the system and increase the time that providers treasure caring for patients and families – that is, building meaningful relationships in order to improve a patient's overall health and well-being.

Taking the long view toward change in a complex setting helps in coping with these changes. Although necessary changes seem difficult at the time of implementation, the adaptations that occur can result in dramatic improvements to the system as a whole. How we manage that change and leverage those changes to improve patient outcomes, system performance, and professional development will be our collective challenge in the future.

References

1. Glouberman S, Zimmerman B. *Complicated and Complex Systems: what would successful reform of Medicare look like?* Discussion Paper No. 8. Commission on the Future of Health Care in Canada; July, 2002.
2. Zimmerman B, Lindberg C, Plsek P. A complexity science primer. In: Zimmerman B, Lindberg C, Plsek PE. *Edgeware: insights from complexity science for health care leaders.* Irving, TX: VHA; 2001. pp. 3–20.
3. Ammenwerth E, Schnell-Inderst P, Machan C, *et al.* The effect of electronic prescribing on medication errors and adverse drug events: a systematic review. *J Am Med Inform Assoc.* 2008; **15**(5): 585–600.
4. Kaushal R, Shojania KG, Bates DW. Effects of computerized physician order entry and clinical decision support systems on medication safety: a systematic review. *Arch Intern Med.* 2003; **163**(12): 1409–16.
5. Wolfstadt JI, Gurwitz JH, Field TS, *et al.* The effect of computerized physician order entry with clinical decision support on the rates of adverse drug events: a systematic review. *J Gen Intern Med.* 2008; **23**(4): 451–8.
6. Wyne K. Information technology for the treatment of diabetes: improving outcomes and controlling cost. *J Manag Care Pharm.* 2008; **14**(2 Suppl.): S12–17.
7. Shekelle PG, Morton SC, Keeler EB. *Costs and Benefits of Health Information Technology.* Evidence Report/Technology Assessment No. 132. (Prepared by the Southern California Evidence-based Practice Center under Contract No. 290-02-0003.) AHRQ Publication No. 06-E006. Rockville, MD: Agency for Healthcare Research and Quality; April 2006.
8. Mitchell M. *Complexity: a guided tour.* Oxford: Oxford University Press; 2009. pp.12–13.
9. Liu S, Prior E, Warren C, *et al.* Improving the quality of care for the hospitalized tobacco user: one institution's transformational journey. *J Cancer Educ.* 2010; **25**(3): 297–301.
10. Hansen LO, Young RS, Hinami K, *et al.* Interventions to reduce 30-day rehospitalisation: a systematic review. *Ann Int Med.* 2011; **155**(8): 520–8.
11. Nuckols TK, Bhattacharya J, Wolman DM, *et al.* Cost implications of reduced work hours and workloads for resident physicians. *N Engl J Med.* 2009; **360**(21): 2202–15.

7

Faculty as Coaches
Their Development and Their Work

Kathryn B. Kirkland and Gautham Suresh

At one corner of the triangle that appears and reappears throughout this book are three words, "better professional development," emphasizing the importance of fostering the development of the health professionals who strive to improve systems of care and patient outcomes. In our Leadership Preventive Medicine Residency (LPMR, described in Chapter 5 of this volume) a key method we use to foster such health professional development is coaching, a dyadic relationship where a faculty member works closely with a resident over the course of 2 years, guiding her in the planning, implementation, and refinement of a health-care improvement project. The lines that connect the triangle's corners and form a reflective space in the center represent the coaching relationship.

In this chapter, we describe our coaching program. Drawing on our experience, and some of the literature on coaching and related topics[1-3] and using case vignettes based on actual coaching experiences (modified to preserve confidentiality), we describe principles and methods to make coaching more effective and the pitfalls to avoid. These principles and methods can be used and adapted in a variety of settings to develop and sustain health professionals who seek to improve health care.

Coaching: Etymology and Vision

The term "coaching," long used in sports, has gained expanded use in recent years, as in executive coaching, life coaching, team building outside of sports, and to apprenticeship/master-teacher models. The etymology of the term suggests "a means of assistance in journeying, transport." It is derived from "Koj," a Hungarian city where vehicles that conveyed people and materials from one place to another were made. We see coaches and coaching as a means of assisting residents in their transformative journeys to become leaders of health-care improvement.

Before discussing our experience in greater detail, it is useful to consider some of the traditional types of health-care faculty-trainee relationships and their features to better understand how we see "coaching" as similar to or different from them.

Faculty-Trainee Relationships in Clinical Training

Though our experience is in medicine, we recognize dyadic relationships between an experienced senior faculty member, clinician, or administrator and a novice, a learner, or a trainee in most health professions and commonly found in both academic and nonacademic health-care institutions. These relationships take many forms – teacher-student, mentor-mentee, advisor-advisee, research guide-doctoral student, coach-"team member," supervisor-supervisee, manager-employee. These dyadic relationships often share the following features:

- a helping person
- a person being helped
- periodic meaningful interactions between them
- transfer of knowledge, information, guidance and advice ("help")
- focus on improving behavior/performance of the person being helped.

We find coaching to be much more deeply involved than most other dyadic faculty-learner relationships. A significant time commitment by both coach and resident learner is required. Beyond time alone, coaching draws on the deepest parts of both professionals, requiring a mutual commitment to learning, discovery and performance improvement. In most other faculty-learner relationships, the more senior member imparts knowledge or a skill to the more junior partner. Although effective mentoring relationships facilitate a learner's independent discovery of knowledge or a skill, a process that often serves to expand the mentor's own understanding and wisdom, we believe that coaching relationships create more evenly balanced partnerships, allowing both participants to move well beyond the preexisting knowledge realm of the coach. In fact, in the coaching relationships we have experienced, the specific knowledge or skill needed to address a particular challenge is often not known a priori by either party, but emerges in the relationship, as the coach asks questions, prompts reflection, or creates time and space during which a subject, a problem, a success or a failure can be explored. A key characteristic of the coaching relationship is this process of co-discovery. The relationship is bilateral, bidirectional, and simultaneous: both participants are likely to grow professionally through the relationship, developing deeper understanding of a shared subject. Coach and resident may walk away from a session with different discoveries, relevant to the different contexts in which they work. Coaching can also provide a safe space for the resident to reflect on personal frustrations and challenges with the improvement work, with the LPMR program, and with maintaining motivation and good spirit. Often these conversations bring insights and ideas worth trying in the effort to learn how to lead change.

The Coaching Arrangement

A coaching relationship, in which a LPM resident is paired with a faculty member experienced in leading health-care improvement, is central to the resident's experience. Although early in the program, pairings were matched by specialty, current coach/resident pairs often cross specialties. For example, an internal medicine resident is matched with a thoracic surgeon, or an infectious disease fellow with a neonatologist. From the beginning of the residency the coach and the resident meet regularly. The coach guides the resident in selecting a practicum, an experience leading change for the improvement of health care in a specific area, building an improvement team within the microsystem, gaining buy-in from microsystem staff, facing organizational barriers, identifying facilitating factors, developing measures for the improvement effort, implementing the improvement through empirical Plan-Do-Study-Act cycles, and writing a scholarly paper about the experience.

The coach is a consistent presence, playing different roles: sometimes a mentor, sometimes a technical advisor, a personal advisor, or a cheerleader for the resident. Through this relationship the coach fosters the development of the "leader within" the resident, by asking questions and promoting reflection on the experience of leading change. "Microsystem mentors" – faculty members from the unit or department in which the improvement project is being done – serve as content experts and local resources for residents. In addition to regular one-on-one meetings, coaches and residents meet formally in group settings with other coaches and residents. Frequently this occurs in work rounds, during which the group reviews work-in-progress. In addition, a coach-resident dyad sometimes meets together with either a microsystem mentor or another member of the LPMR faculty with expertise in measurement, a particular methodology, or another specific knowledge domain.

The Role of a "Third Thing" Linking Coach and Resident

Parker Palmer[4] describes the role of "third things," elements that serve as a provocation for or an indirect embodiment of an important topic for a group to address, but which may be too threatening if faced directly. He describes poems, artwork, stories which reveal important truths in an oblique, or metaphorical, way. For us, the regular meetings between coach and resident also involve a "third thing," an element other than coach or resident that threads through the development of their relationship, serving as substrate for reflective conversation about the practice of leading change. It is unusual for resident and coach to have a discussion specifically about the topic of leadership when they meet. Instead the meetings often focus on a third thing, the actual work of the resident (and sometimes of the coach too), concrete events that allow consideration of the leadership of health-care improvement. In contrast to Palmer's third thing, a metaphor that allows discussion of the concrete, the third thing for coaching the development of leadership is the change-work itself, with all of its concrete and specific challenges, struggles, and successes. The discussion of the work precipitates questions and conversation between coach and resident about the nature of leadership. What does it take to be an effective leader? What are the barriers to change? How does one work with multidisciplinary teams, in different contexts, to facilitate change? What counts as improvement? How do we know we have achieved it? What can we learn from failure?

Reflection on this third thing, the change-work, and the varied forms it takes as residents and coaches dive into the specifics of the improvement projects at hand, provide the structure within which the coaching relationship develops. The questions that emerge – often compelling to the improvement work of both coach and resident – prompt professional growth and reflection for both. The struggles of the resident often mirror those of the coach. The successes resonate; the failures feel familiar. Every 2–3 weeks, two people gather to explore the concrete events, reflecting on them together, identifying the questions, and working collaboratively to discover answers, to plan next steps, to celebrate small successes and to dissect failures. Both leave with new understanding that helps them in their work. As coaches, we have often taken more from a coaching session than the resident. Even as we experience the pleasure of helping a resident understand a meeting gone awry, or an uncomfortable interaction, we also gain new ideas and insights into our own work. This two-layered process, regularly repeated, sustains us as humans, creating a sense of empowerment and, at times joy, about our own ongoing efforts to improve systems and achieve better outcomes for patients. The residents report a similar benefit.

Preparing to be a Coach

Some faculty members may be naturally more adept at coaching than others, but all can benefit from developing and mastering a set of skills, and from reflecting on their efforts at coaching. Based on our experience, several competencies are required for successful coaching:

- the ability to develop and nurture a relationship that will facilitate growth in the learner, through customizing it as required by the specific characteristics and requirements of the learner
- reflective listening skills and ongoing personal reflective practice
- the ability to guide the learner in self-reflection
- the ability to understand the learner's level of knowledge, personality, time-management skills, social skills, strengths and weaknesses
- a willingness to engage in understanding aspects of the learner's personal life that might affect his or her performance at work (e.g., a wife's pregnancy or an impending specialty board examination)
- the ability to monitor the learner's progress through the experiential learning of the project and guide the learner's course while not being too authoritarian or intrusive or prescriptive, and allowing the learner to learn from his or her own mistakes.

Additional coaching skills in our residency program relate to health care improvement, often developed through the coach's own experience in the leadership of improvement:

- improvement content expertise: how to develop a global and specific aim, how to map a process, how to identify change concepts and theories of improvement, how to measure the results of tests of change, and how to identify and subsequently contextualize generalizable scientific knowledge
- project management skills: how to organize a project, identify project milestones, and monitor whether or not a project is on track
- knowledge of human psychology and group dynamics
- an understanding of the organizational and system context where the learner will be attempting to conduct the test of change, including the organization's financial and management conditions, politics, pressures, priorities, constraints, and the forces buffeting the organization and their potential effect(s) on the learner's project.

Frames of Understanding
••••••••••••••••••••••••••••••

Although the knowledge and skills above are helpful in preparing to be a coach, we have learned that the process of coaching cannot be reduced to a set of linear tasks, or a checklist of behaviors. We have learned that we need to understand the ways in which residents understand and assign meaning to their experiences. Effective coaching starts with careful listening to the language used by a resident to describe the way they are making sense of what they notice. The language and the frames used can limit what is recognized. By expanding their language, a coach can introduce alternate views that may enable a resident to see and achieve a different outcome. Just as every system is designed to get the results it gets, so every resident's view of the world may restrict them to seeing only certain options and outcomes. Effective leadership of change can require new ways of seeing, speaking, and doing. Modeling this, the coach can provide a different perspective, and introduce new language for new insight and understanding. By encouraging the resident to test these new ways, a coach can facilitate the development of self-correcting and self-generating approaches to leading change. Likewise, sometimes the resident's view as "new eyes on the ground," can transform a coach's view allowing him or her to develop new language for characterizing problems and proposed solutions.

Preparing to be Coached: The Learner
•••

Residents can prepare themselves for a good coaching experience, just as coaches can prepare and develop themselves. Our residents enter from clinical residencies, which mostly emphasize domains of knowledge and skills not directly related to the work necessary to lead local organizational change for the improvement of health care. Few of our residents starting the program are skilled in leading change, or in working within a long-term coaching relationship; some may even resist developing new skills when the previous clinical habits have worked well. An early explicit discussion of what the resident can do that will enhance the effectiveness of the coaching relationship can help and this may include:

- a willingness to seek guidance and an openness to "shaping" through a relationship with an assigned coach – that is, a willingness to submit to being coached
- a willingness to balance independent self-driven work and planning with openness to learning and modifying plans arising from coaching sessions
- commitment to meet with the coach on a regular basis
- a commitment to preparing for coaching sessions to maximize the productivity of this time (requires skill in summarizing activities and progress and

identifying areas where help is needed, framing questions for discussion, reflection)

- good listening skills
- an openness to and even eagerness for questions, input, and feedback (including constructive negative feedback) with the ability to react to it without demonstrating defensiveness, denial or deflection
- a commitment to regular reflection related to health-care improvement activities, leadership development, and other relevant issues that emerge during coaching sessions.

The Coaching Journey

A coach who comes to the relationship desiring to foster a nurturing long-term relationship, the ability to listen reflectively, and the knowledge, skill, and experience of leading the improvement of health care can help create a fertile environment for a resident to explore what it means to lead improvement. Similarly, a resident who arrives with enthusiasm for the work, receptivity to the open-ended nature of the coaching relationship, and a willingness to practice active reflection enhances the likelihood of creating an environment in which the relationship and mutual learning will thrive. From the beginning, the coach and resident share responsibility for the relationship they will create, and the ways in which each will benefit.

Although the 2-year coaching relationship develops iteratively and is in many ways unique to the individuals who create it, we think that certain stages or phases have been commonly observed across different dyads. These include explicit setting of aims and commitment to mutual work, co-creation of a set of expectations for one another, assessment of strengths, weaknesses, and skills of the resident, relationship development, and awareness of and reaction to specific events that serve as openings for learning, reflection and coaching. In our experience, these phases do not occur in a linear way, but may thread through the entire journey, weaving together in different ways for different coach-resident pairs. For instance, setting aims and expectations, which often occurs at the initial phase of a journey, may be revisited at intervals throughout the entire residency, as new challenges and contexts develop.

Setting Aims and Expectations

When the coach and resident first meet, we have found that it is helpful for them to discuss their concepts of what coaching means, what outcomes are expected, the expectations that each has of the other, and any special constraints (e.g., availability for meetings) or needs (e.g., lack of confidence with writing skills for the learner, or the need to improve time-management skills) each may have. Early in this stage identifying the qualities and skills that resident and coach can develop and bring to the shared work can help. In our program, the coach has had experience with previous coaching relationships. The resident, however, is almost always new to this way of working and so there is a need to prepare for the most productive way of working in this way.

A critical step involves the explicit discussion of intended outcomes, and the resident and coach commitments to creating them. Working from implicit presumptions that the work underway is in service of shared outcomes can lead to mistakes, misunderstandings, and wasted time. Common mistakes during the early relationship include assuming a level of commitment the resident does not yet have, acting as if no commitment is required of the coach, and failing to articulate the intended outcomes, and the potential obstacles to their realization. In discussions about these issues, openness, honesty, and completeness are essential. Lively and active dialogue is required between coach and resident about the specific context of the work, the uncertainties of the future, and the limitations and strengths of both participants.

Assessment

A second theme, which threads through the 2 years, is assessment. The coach develops a deep understanding of the resident's strengths and weaknesses, skills, and ways of interpreting the world and its events. Much of this understanding develops through listening to the resident describe her work, the challenges encountered, and the resident's responses to them. There is a role, too, for gaining knowledge of personal aspects of a resident's life that may influence her way of approaching her work, or enhance or limit her effectiveness. Finding ways to share these insights in ways that allow the resident to benefit from the feedback is key.

Attention to "Openings"

Coaching begins in earnest when specific or "triggering" events occur. Flaherty calls these events "openings" and this seems an apt metaphor to us.[1] When a routine is disturbed or an unusual or unexpected event occurs, such as something breaking down, an unanticipated reorganization, or a change in circumstance that requires a new skill offer an opening for conversation. In our residents' practicum work, openings occur when they face unexpected barriers to improvement, feel overwhelmed by the scope of the work, first launch their improvement project, participate in regularly scheduled work rounds, and before major formal presentations to the Practicum Review Board of senior health system leaders. Recently residents have experienced "openings" associated with implementation of a new electronic medical record, and loss of some senior members of their improvement teams related to early retirement. While these events initially appear disruptive and unsettling, they can present wonderful opportunities for learning important leadership lessons. Often it is the coach who sees the learning value of the disruption, but sometimes, a resident will be the one to recognize the need to bring forward the unexpected experience for discussion and mutual exploration.

Relationship

As we have repeatedly experienced, the foundation for this faculty role of coaching is found in the relationship between the coach and learner. The development of this relationship is crucial and cannot be assumed, neglected or considered unnecessary. We agree with Flaherty[1] that mutual trust, respect, and freedom of expression are essential. We believe that these factors more than the presence of "chemistry," mutual liking or even shared interests and experiences actually facilitate the development of a successful coaching relationship. In our program, cross-disciplinary coaching relationships have been built intentionally through openness, communication, appreciation, fairness, and shared commitment. Some regard these assigned coach-resident pairings as a form of an arranged marriage. A match is made, and with mutual investment of time and commitment, a unique and durable relationship grows. Without explicit investment in creating the relationship, it is unlikely to serve as the foundation for a rich and productive life.

The Work and Benefits of Coaching

We have learned that it is preferable to have regularly scheduled meetings between the coach and the learner. During the beginning of the project these meetings should ideally occur at least once in two weeks or more frequently. In addition to these regular meetings, the coach should be available to meet with the learner when special situations arise, as when the resident encounters an unanticipated barrier. Brief minutes of the meetings can be kept, so that both coach and learner can look back and refresh their memories as needed about the discussions they have had. Alternatively the coach and resident might keep their own notes about the sessions, and compare them periodically. It is often helpful for the coach to visit the setting where the resident is carrying out the improvement work so that a deeper understanding of the context of the improvement work can be developed. The coach's different perspective may allow the resident to view events and their meaning differently, opening up new understanding and ideas for actions that can help address barriers that have arisen. Coaches who have learned to offer insights in the form of questions have seen residents create their own interpretations, rather than simply receive a coach's advice. As coaches have often served in other faculty roles, they need to be wary of slipping into roles that may be more familiar or comfortable – such as a teacher, or supervisor, roles that may encourage more passive learning on the part of the resident.

A residency with a long-term coaching relationship at its center was formed as a way to facilitate the formation of young professionals as they experientially developed the knowledge and skill to become leaders of the improvement of health care. What has become clear to the coaches, as they have served in this role, is that the relationship is equally beneficial for them. As the following representative coaching stories illustrate, the challenges faced by residents often mirror those of the coaches. Through a process of co-discovery, a coach often leaves a coaching session with new ideas about how to approach her own improvement aim. By sharing and reflecting on coaching experiences among fellow coaches at regularly scheduled faculty development meetings, our group of faculty coaches has created a kind of "community of practice,"[5,6] contributing to our own development and a deeper understanding of our role in sustaining people capable of leading the improvement of health care into the future. Eight years into our coaching program we submit that in addition to training residents to be leaders in health-care improvement, coaching may be a key to sustaining the similar work of the coaches themselves, who are typically older and more experienced in this world, but who similarly need to nurture themselves in order to receive joy and renewed commitment to their work.

These stories depict the experiences of several different resident-coach dyads and illustrate the way in which the professional developmental journeys of coach and resident intertwine as they seek to improve health care and to learn how to do this more effectively within a mutually supportive, mutually beneficial learning relationship. They also serve as powerful illustrations of the importance of each component of the triangle, and the ways in which the corners are linked and mutually supportive of the whole. All the stories are written from the coach's perspective, reflecting events as seen by a coach or coaches.

Understanding Coaching: Stories from Real Life

Coaching George: George's story illustrates the parallels between the leadership journeys of coach and resident and the ways in which unexpected events can be used in coaching to promote reflection and learning in both.

George is a slightly disorganized, likeable infectious diseases fellow and leadership preventive medicine resident. I serve as his coach. George has a huge heart and a big presence. He is in a bit of a pickle, and it's a pickle that is pretty familiar to me.

Each resident chooses a year-long project in clinical improvement as a major element of experiential learning about leading change in their training in the residency. They "try out" the leadership and health-care improvement skills they have learned through classes, smaller projects, and coaching sessions. George wants to improve hand hygiene, and has chosen the hospital unit that has the lowest observed hand hygiene rates: 10%. As part of his initial assessment he has administered a survey to the staff of this unit to assess their "readiness for change." They are not ready; in fact they are "pre-contemplative" in the Prochaska typology.[7] When his proposal was up for review by the group of senior leaders who approve resident improvement projects, they legitimately questioned the allocation of resources to a project that is likely to fail, sending George back to have further conversations with his coach to develop a Plan B.

He and I sit together in my office, considering the situation. It is true that the unit staff does not yet realize they have a problem – a common situation in my world of infection prevention! But it is also true that this unit is missing 90% of hand hygiene opportunities, a situation that feels difficult to walk away from. How can we begin a project in a unit that is "not ready"? How can we not? The dilemma leads us to more questions. How might we help the unit become more ready for change? Is it possible that the initiation of improvement work itself could lead to better receptivity to that same improvement? Is testing this hypothesis justifiable? Should we move the project to another unit, with staff who are more receptive to change (but less in need of it)? We remind ourselves of the goals of the resident project: we seek not just to improve health care but to learn something about leading in this domain – through successes but also through failures if they occur. George's project gradually reemerges as an experiment in implementing change in an environment that is unreceptive, and possibly even hostile to the concept. It is clear to me that lessons we will learn through this work have the potential to yield major benefit for me in my own work, and for others at our medical center. We frame a plan for moving forward which George presents successfully to the review board the following week.

I look back on this coaching conversation now with the benefit of several years of hindsight. George has long since moved on to other venues, but the hand hygiene improvement that occurred in this low-performing unit that was unready for change has lasted through those years. Through trial and error, George learned that improvement in this context required a deep understanding of the actual work processes in this very busy unit, and the insertion of a hand sanitizer at a point that made its use a natural part of the workflow. I learned an enormously important lesson that acceptance of the need for improvement is not an absolute prerequisite to beginning improvement work, and that in fact, acceptance of change can be a result of measured improvement. A second staff survey administered toward the end of his yearlong project revealed a major shift in the stage of change reflected by unit staff.

I still see George at national meetings and reflect with him on the work we did together, those moments of dismay that the project would have to be scrapped, the discouraging results of efforts to educate and market the need for hand hygiene to the staff, the gradual understanding of the need to see the work itself, and the elation of measured improvement as it emerged on the statistical process control charts. Then we share stories of improvement work we continue to do, much of which builds on and further confirms the lessons learned during his practicum year, and some of which continue to surprise.

Coaching Sara: Sara's story highlights the ways in which questions posed by a coach can elucidate a resident's current way of seeing and sense-making, allowing the resident to develop new insights into how she finds meaning in events, and then to make deliberate changes in how she chooses to see and approach a situation.

Sara is upset. She has come from a meeting with Janet, another faculty member with expertise in data analysis, during which they were to review her data and the charts she has constructed to illustrate responses to a series of planned and unplanned interventions designed to improve the timely delivery of antibiotics to inpatients on the medical service. She has been excited to see evidence of improvement. But Janet has suggested that Sara's approach to the data is not appropriate; moreover, she has apparently failed to understand or accept Sara's rationale for doing it the way she has. Sara is deflated and outraged. I lean back in my chair and listen while Sara delineates the many ways in which the faculty member has fallen short: she describes her lack of understanding, her inability to listen or flex with the situation; she questions the validity of her knowledge and advice, citing a different perspective provided by a more senior faculty member; she eventually closes by pronouncing Janet unable to work effectively with residents and stating her own unwillingness to meet with her again. She stops and looks at me, her coach, for a response. I let the silence create a space for reflection.

I am thinking about what Sara has said. I know Sara's data and believe that the way she has approached the analysis is rational. I have worked with Janet over the years and have found her to provide a very useful perspective for the residents and for me. Like Sara, I have noticed that Janet's approach is occasionally inflexible, and that she can be quite concrete. I have also noticed her tendency to become more rigid and less able to communicate in situations that become confrontational or polarized, and I suspect this is what has happened in the just concluded meeting.

I am also thinking about who Sara is, and her development as a leader. Sara is an energetic, engaging, and impatient woman with exacting standards for herself and others and an unwavering commitment to improving health care. Sara is a strong clinician and open to learning; she has worked well in facilitating the development of a team that is engaged in designing the tests of change that have been implemented. I know Sara well enough to be aware that she has little tolerance for others who fall short in her eyes; when she becomes impatient, it is easy for others to see. I can imagine her demeanor in the meeting.

I pause, look at Sara and pose a question: "In what ways do you think you and Janet might be similar?" She looks back at me, off balance from the question, which was not what she was expecting. "We're nothing alike," she responds. "I don't understand what you are saying." I offer that I have worked with both of them over several years and that I think there are some similarities in how they may deal with differences of opinion, and with conflict. "Think about what you are bringing to a meeting like this. What are your expectations? How well are you anticipating and preparing for the range of responses you may encounter? How do you understand Janet and what she will bring? How are you showing up for her?" She looks at me, speechless, as I continue. "You want to lead improvement, right? So how are you going to learn from this situation? Go think about it, write about it, and see what you come up with."

How many times have I had meetings that didn't go as planned, in which my carefully planned agendas didn't play out, when other people had opinions that slowed me down, introduced complexity, or pushed my buttons? I think about the ways in which I tend to meet the resistance of others with my own resistance, polarizing issues instead of seeking the "both-and" solutions. I think about the ways I might be dismissive of opinions that didn't align with mine, and the ways in which all of these responses slowed down improvement rather than speeding it up. How am I showing up for people in these situations and how might I want to choose to change that, in the interest of our shared aims?

Sara returns the following week, brimming with fresh insights, gained from her own writing and reflection. We talk about the ways in which both Sara and Janet tend to dig in their heels in the face of conflict, clinging even harder to their preconceived positions the more obvious it becomes that listening and creativity is what is needed. Sara asserts that as a leader she needs to figure out how to overcome the challenges posed by this kind of dynamic. She has thought through the various drivers of the last meeting's dysfunctional outcome and has ideas for a few small tests of change to try. She has shifted from seeing Janet as the problem, or even herself as the problem, to focusing on using her knowledge of process improvement to create an environment where a different outcome is more likely. She admits, "You really shocked me when you said we were alike, but after I thought about it, I realized you were right!"

Two years later, Sara serves as a leader in a large organization, a role that requires her to manage the candid, impatient, and even impulsive aspects of her personality. She periodically reports on politically charged encounters that she is proud of having navigated, and speaks of the importance of reflecting about the person she is bringing to the conversations. As I continue to help resolve power struggles that subsequent residents and even I occasionally become engaged in, this conversation with Sara often serves as a touchstone for me. The coaching relationship creates a space where residents and coaches can work on themselves, asking critical questions about what leadership is, and how leaders invite a range of opinions and ideas that together lead to changes that build better systems and achieve better outcomes for patients.

Coaching Anthony: Anthony's story illustrates the value of the work and reflection that takes place outside of a session, in the context of the improvement work being done by both resident and coach.

I open the e-mail and read, with dismay, the problem for which Anthony is seeking my help. His current challenge almost exactly mirrors one that I am struggling with in my own work. How does one react when, in the process of trying to "lead change" one encounters others, necessary to the work, who choose not to engage, who seem to offer impediments rather than collaboration? Anthony spells out the situation, and he offers a list of responses he is considering, for my reaction. I close the e-mail with the thought: I can't help Anthony on this one; I don't know the right answer myself.

Anthony, a resident in his second year, has been trying to get his team together to begin working on their first intervention aimed at improving clinic access for patients. He and his team want to bring in a patient adviser to join the group, to help keep the patient experience at the center. His department director wants to wait, isn't so sure this is a good idea, and expects pushback from other department members who are not members of the improvement team. She has offered a series of things that need to happen before she can feel comfortable going ahead with the meeting. Anthony feels paralyzed, and frustrated that he is now unable to move forward because he has tried to include her, and has received a directive, not a collaborative response.

I am struggling with a similar challenge as I try to get engagement from a group of surgeons and perioperative leaders who I believe share responsibility for several patients who have developed infections following surgical procedures. The responses I have received range from no response at all to indications that it will be weeks before they will have time for a meeting, to suggestions about what "I" should do next to solve "my" problem. I want them to engage with me so that we can work on the problem as a team. I am not getting a directive response, but it isn't collaborative either.

As I contemplate the parallel nature of our current challenges, I begin to anticipate our meeting: this will be an opportunity for me to learn something about what to do next, even as I try to help Anthony develop a plan.

When Anthony and I meet we begin by trying to name the things that might be going on when someone stalls, delays, or undermines progress. We consider the various ways in which we might unwittingly precipitate such undesired reactions. Do we sometimes take an approach that is too direct when an oblique one might work better? Do we lay out options that appear too black and white (possibly because of our own preconceived notions about which path will lead to success)? Do we choose to "ask for permission" when it might work better to "keep informed," or "invite to contribute"? We even consider methods of communication: is e-mail as effective a tool as a phone call or a face-to-face conversation for engaging others? It isn't clear to either of us whether our way of approaching others has contributed to the results that we are getting, but we both benefit from the opportunity these questions create to reflect on the possibility. As we consider them, we become aware that there are often a variety of ways to get where one wants to go, and recognize a tendency that we share to stay fixed on the one "right way" that has occurred to us. Both of us leave the meeting with ideas of what to try next.

As we reflect on these, and other coaching journeys we have shared with residents in our program, we are very aware of the space that this developing relationship creates and occupies in the world of health-care improvement. As we consider coaching in the context of the triangle, perhaps the coaching relationship could also be seen as the "space" in the center of the triangle, a space for learning and reflection. The ultimate aim of both resident and coach is better outcomes for individuals and for populations of patients. The way they try to achieve this aim is through understanding the system that holds the current situation in place, and which can be changed to yield the desired situation; they use time, space, and relationship, to reflect and learn at every step, nurturing the formation and the development of professionals who find meaning, and even joy, in this work.

All health care is ultimately delivered to individual human beings by other human beings, working together to provide the best care possible. Attention to the formation, development, and sustenance of humans who are involved in this health care delivery is critical. Yet, in a world increasingly focused on quantitative measures, and best practices, the human element seems in danger of being overlooked. By establishing the place of a specific relationship at the center of the improvement triangle we take a step toward formalizing the centrality of people, everyone, to all health care delivery.

While this chapter has focused on coaching in the context of the residents and faculty of a specific residency program designed to develop leaders of health care improvement, we believe that a focus on relationships as the space within which professionals learn, reflect, grow, and improve, has wide applicability within all of health care. Coaching relationships likely exist in many forms already, but unless we name them and insist upon them, we risk losing an appreciation of their importance. "Third things" that could, and in some cases already do, inform the substrate for such relationships abound: themes of teamwork, communication, decision making, prioritization thread through many areas of health care, as do people who work in health care, in every discipline, and at every level from novice to expert. We believe that strengthening coaching relationships and integrating them into the ongoing professional formation that is central to all good health care delivery, beginning with medical, nursing, and other students and continuing through the development of graduate level professionals and those who continue to learn and develop throughout their careers connects people with each other in ways that ensure that the enterprise reflected in the model of the whole triangle remains sturdy enough to allow sustained work to improve systems and improve outcomes and experiences of patients.

References

1. Flaherty J. *Coaching: evoking excellence in others*. 3rd ed. Burlington, MA: Butterworth-Heinemann; 2010.
2. Schein E. *Helping*. San Francisco, CA: Berrett-Koehler; 2009.
3. Gawande A. Personal best. *New Yorker*. October 3, 2011.
4. Palmer P. *A Hidden Wholeness: the journey toward an undivided life*. San Francisco, CA: Jossey-Bass; 2004.
5. Lave J, Wenger E. *Situated Learning: legitimate peripheral participation*. Cambridge: Cambridge University Press; 1991.
6. Wenger E. *Communities of Practice*. New York, NY: Cambridge University Press; 2000.
7. Prochaska JO. Decision making in the transtheoretical model of behavior change. *Med Decis Making*. 2008; **28**(6): 845–9.

8

Governance, Leadership, Management, Organizational Structure, and Oversight Principles and Practices

James Anderson

Late in 2010 one of our most renowned surgeons, Robin Cotton, MD, sent me a note on my retirement as chief executive officer (CEO) of Cincinnati Children's Hospital Medical Center, recounting that during his first 20 years he was able to build an internationally recognized department because of *individual* effort and a permissive institution; during the last 10 he was able to build the department because of the *institution*.

His experience demonstrates the impact of Cincinnati Children's new commitment to dramatically improving the health care delivery system and our organizational performance. The results have been felt across the interdependent triangle of better patient outcomes, operational excellence, and professional development, made possible by a system characterized by a deliberately integrated effort among caregivers, patients, and support systems. We have learned that we all operate in a highly complex, interdependent system that can only deliver the best health results if every part operates at nothing short of excellence.

Our experience at Cincinnati Children's teaches a valuable lesson: "When every part operates excellently, our patients are healthier, we consume fewer resources and we deliver better results. Our sense of obligation and generosity to each other grows as our dependence on each other becomes clearer and we develop professionally to sustain these results."

How did this profound transformation – as yet incomplete – happen? There were a number of influencing, encouraging events that led to commitment to transformation, but the triggering event was associated with this same surgeon, who came to Cincinnati as a result of getting onto the wrong airplane in 1972, not having funds to go further and happening to know a fellow ear, nose, and throat (ENT) surgeon in Cincinnati who took him in.

The triggering event occurred while we were developing the institution's first strategic plan under new rules inviting broadly based deep and boundary-less thinking on the subject of what Cincinnati Children's needed to do during the next five years to pursue its vision "to be the leader in improving child health." Our board of trustees had adopted that vision in 1996 after 2 years of discussion. I was chairman of the board at the time. We all recognized that the institution was not yet that leader, and that to achieve our vision would require constant change, investment, and improvement to take our organizational performance and our impact on child health to unprecedented levels of excellence.

Against that backdrop in 2001, senior management asked several clinical teams what Cincinnati Children's must achieve to advance against our newly articulated vision. Our restless ENT surgeon co-chaired the group asked to outline a path forward for ambulatory care. On behalf of his co-chair and team, he simply stated that the systems relied upon to deliver care were so dysfunctional, required so many workarounds and were so inefficient that until the institution fixed those, its ability to dramatically improve ambulatory care or any other care would be severely impaired. The message was: The institution needs to commit to and deliver operational excellence. Without it, improved care is unachievable. He asserted the linkage between operational excellence and improved patient outcomes.

Other events supported Cincinnati Children's interest in transformation. In discussions about our new vision, trustees agreed our high potential to deliver better pediatric health was unrealized. We celebrated pockets of excellence but recognized the institution hadn't figured out how to deliver excellence as a reliable product of its activities. Why were we delivering spectacular results (e.g., the Sabin oral polio vaccine) occasionally but undistinguished results mostly? Did we really know what results we were delivering? How were we measuring results? If we were capable of delivering noteworthy results in some areas, why not all areas? The institution was strong financially, had a strong market position, strong community support, well developed clinical and research infrastructures – all the big pieces needed to excel broadly. Yet it wasn't. The problem must be us. The board should expect more and provide the support needed for rapid evolution. The time was ripe to take the institution to the next level – wherever that might be.

It was also clear that none of us knew what that next level looked like or exactly how to get there. As board chair I was convinced of our under-realized potential, the strength of our resources and the support of the board for open-minded, thoughtful pursuit of our bold new vision. I was convinced that if we got the vision right – and I believed after two years of discussion we did – we were capable of taking bold steps. We just needed to figure out what they would be.

Seeking a Change Agent

Fortuitously, during the period we were finalizing our vision, we were also engaged in a national search for a new chief executive officer (CEO). As we advanced our thinking as a board through open discussion about our vision for the institution, we also were advancing our thinking about what we would need in a new CEO. Imperceptibly, as we gained comfort and courage about the radical nature of our vision, our minds opened as to the kind of CEO we would need to take us there.

Our search was conventionally organized. As board chair, I had appointed a diverse senior search committee, retained a nationally known search firm and appointed myself chair of the committee. We began the process with more than 100 interviews by the search firm to develop a broad sense of what characteristics our new CEO should have. As the results of the interviews came in and candidates began to be considered, more energy developed behind bold pursuit of our new vision.

Increasingly, the search committee doubted that a conventional candidate whose experience was limited to the health care culture would be successful in leading the radical change contemplated by our vision. During this period of intimately considering the implications of our vision and the opportunity to pick a leader to deliver it, expectations rose and the willingness to consider unconventional change agents as CEO blossomed.

The end result, after a series of meetings of which I had no knowledge, was that – to my surprise – the search committee offered the CEO position to me, a lawyer who had experience in a manufacturing company and who had been a board member for almost 20 years. After some thought and consultation, I accepted the unexpected offer and became CEO on November 1, 1996.

At the same moment, newly and unexpectedly in need of a board chair, the committee offered the position to Lee Carter, a longtime board member and generous community leader with a consumer marketing background. The two of us, friends and coworkers for decades on various community projects, set about to shape the future of Cincinnati Children's.

Planning for Bold Action

We were free of knowledge of how health care actually worked and of its traditional operating practices. We were energized, open-minded and very much wanted to make a difference, to have an impact on child health. Lee was particularly imaginative and creative. We had the newly embraced vision. We had inherited an organization that had recruited physicians and scientists well, had built a prominent research program and had expanded its programs and facilities significantly. Building on that now we had the opportunity and obligation to deliver the new vision.

Privately we wondered together about what limits the board might have on what we initiated. They had given us the job, but what did they really want, and how much adventure would they support? During an impromptu conversation we had with a board leader about what she thought we could do, she glanced away, shook her head, and said, "Why, I think you can do anything you want." Lee and I looked at each other, nodded and said, "Great. Thanks." That quick conversation removed countless barriers known and unknown and enabled us to pursue the promise of transformation.

We had inherited an institution which for the preceding 15 years had been adding operational infrastructure where none had existed. It was evolving from a loose confederation of physicians who shared an interest in pediatrics and occupied common ground in a facility but whose individual independence was their hallmark to one with more substantial threads to the institution.

The structure had begun evolving out of necessity. Cincinnati Children's could barely make payroll in the mid-1970s and had few systems in place except those essential to employment and necessary to provide staffed beds, operating rooms, and clinics. A crisis meeting the payroll had forced the institution to create a more effective billing system. Financial systems were developed to send hospital bills, a practice not regularly followed until the payroll crisis appeared. Rudimentary budgets followed, and slowly the institution developed tools to manage itself. Significantly these often came at the insistence of trustees who worked in business. Among the physicians, enthusiasm for the new direction was mixed. These new financial and business tools were intrusive, and as likely as not they stimulated protective instincts rather than a heightened sense of opportunity. Supporters, however, among whom was Pediatrics Chair William K. Schubert, MD, who was also our medical center president and CEO, recognized that unless the institution operated effectively, its horizons would be limited.

By 1996, the operating system essentials – including integrated budgeting, financial reporting, system-wide human resources, supply chain management and facilities management – were in place at a basic level and open to improvement. Yet to be developed was the expectation for patient outcomes, operational excellence, and professional development, as well as the tools and metrics to deliver them on a system-wide basis.

In my first days as CEO, as I talked with clinicians and administrators to better understand how the place really worked, it became clear to me that the institution was not organized to be nimble. Opportunities to improve outcomes were not visible to the multiple disciplines that were needed to deliver the improvements. We all desired operational excellence, but the levers to deliver it were not identified or available. When visible, the levers often didn't work.

Their experience often confirmed the doctors' suspicions that the favorable results they achieved were in spite of the efforts of those who administered the system within which they were forced to work. Instead of all sharing the excitement of new advances and of our collective contribution to leadership in improving child health, the staff focused on the hospital's dramatic inadequacies in delivering daily needs. People asked for better workarounds, not for a strategically improved system.

The gaps between our aspirations of leadership and the realities of daily life were severe. Individual cohorts of clinicians and administrators were doing excellent work, but the macrosystem within which they operated made opportunities to lead more difficult, not less. The macrosystem rather than being a source of energy, support, and resources for leadership and excellence was a problem to be overcome. Much as Dr. Cotton pointed out in his note written in 2010, the achievements of his department in those years came as a result of his individual effort, not as a result of the institution.

What I found in my first 60 days was an institution organized in professional channels – physician, nurse, and business – with complete separation of channels until they joined in their common reporting to the CEO. They interacted as needed throughout the organization, but the institution had not structured or supported that interaction in pursuit of institutional goals. Coordinated action happened because it had to or was forced by a strong-willed person trying to avoid bad things and accomplish good things. The tools were few. The sustainability of change was difficult, and there were huge gaps for which no one was accountable.

My experience, all non-health care, preached the wisdom of putting the act of decision making as close as possible to where action occurred in the market. To the extent possible, decisions should be made at the interface between the institution and the customer/client/patient. Individuals in those positions are closest to patients' needs, can see what works and what doesn't, and are the delivery point for operational excellence as well as improved medical outcomes.

Were we organized to capture that intelligence? No. Did we have the mechanisms to respond quickly when change was required? Not likely.

I recall thinking that we were organized to deliver the exact opposite result. Caregivers were isolated, without the tools or resources to solve problems and worse, receiving no message from the institution that outcomes mattered enough to provide those tools and resources. By default, and not intended by top leadership, we had created a culture of "no," in the bowels of the organization.

Imagine a frontline caregiver with an idea that would improve outcomes but required behavior change by someone not in his channel. How would he get it done? Robin Cotton, MD, a division director, could insist on broad-based change and would be successful within his ENT division, but depending on individuals like him to be the sole change agents is neither responsible nor effective. There aren't many like him; their scope is narrow; and the changes they seek may not advance institutional priorities.

A thoughtful and persistent nurse would have to go up her chain of command with her proposed change – an uninviting and sometimes difficult road – and eventually the chief nursing officer might meet with the CEO, surgeon-in-chief, and senior administrative representative to make the case for the CEO to decide. That scenario, while cumbersome, might be plausible with a CEO with strong health care experience, but few would argue that it made any sense with a lawyer/businessman CEO. In truth, that organizational structure cannot deliver the agility necessary for an organization whose vision is to be the leader in improving child health no matter who the leader is.

Not only was the ability to conceive and execute change inhibited by our organizational structure, but our ability to illuminate and spread an improved process also was diminished. There was no effective mechanism to set institutional goals, along with metrics for their achievement, or to connect the essential participants. The channels for advancing integrated action were separated to the highest organizational levels.

I came to the conclusion that if our vision required transformational change, as we believed it did, our organizational structure was profoundly ill-suited to deliver it. Without the ability to execute a shared vision and sustain the changes it required, we could not achieve the radical change the Institute of Medicine envisioned[1,2] and we sought.

As I described what I found to our senior leaders in many conversations, I asked whether this structure made sense. What was I missing? We knew where we wanted to go. How would this structure get us there? No one defended it other than as a product of where we had been. Our vision called for us to leave where we had been and get about the business of improving child health. We needed all the help we could get, including a management structure that would enable that change.

Managing Through Business Units

We decided to create business units covering more than 80% of revenues and a greater percentage of net income. We developed templated financial reports for each business unit as though each were a stand-alone operation. The reports covered 5 years back, the current year, and 3 years forward. Our senior leaders (CEO, chief medical officer, chief nursing officer, chief financial officer, and so forth) met with the leadership of each unit three times a year. The business unit leadership team consisted of the physician division director, nurse unit leader and the division business director. In addition to the financial template, which told the story of the business unit in numbers over a 9-year period, the units were required to use a template form to report progress on other specific institutional objectives, including patient and employee safety, and specific improvement initiatives. Specific focus on market opportunities and the resources needed to deliver results were regular discussion points. At the business unit meetings, financial reports included all revenues generated and costs incurred by the division to deliver its services, including physician costs, nurse costs, administrative costs, heat, light and power, depreciation, malpractice insurance, and the like. Our intention was to provide to everyone a comprehensive picture of the business unit's activity over time, expressed in numbers. It was the first time most had seen such an integrated presentation, and it provided a holistic view of business unit activity as a framework for change. In the course of our meetings and preparation for them, we each learned more about the other's world and what was required to succeed. A "language of the commons" emerged and the professional development of physicians, nurses and administrators advanced at a brisk pace.

The structural elements (senior management participation, template reporting and regular meetings) taken together provided a singular framework to support and manage the execution of our plan, whatever its objectives. Having the senior physician, nurse and business person sharing objectives at a level that directly provides services to patients was a new experience for each and required each to understand the needs of the others in order to succeed in their own objectives. Developing and presenting a single budget for all business unit activity required each to commit sufficient resources to enable the others to achieve their goals. If a physician was adding a new program, nurse staffing had to adjust, and business needs caused by that had to be met. If an initiative to reduce infection were unleashed, each leader had to determine what would be required to reflect that effort in the integrated forecast. Importantly, business unit leadership was often asked to engage families and patients in their planning. Having input from families fostered new understanding, engagement with the initiator and support for an integrated approach. Bringing everyone together, from the frontline caregivers to senior leaders enabled institutional leadership to challenge the entire line of management to identify opportunities for improvement and to present plans to pursue them. For the business units, the chance to present ideas to senior leaders held the promise of access to institutional resources to take advantage of those new opportunities.

Benefits of Template Reporting and Predictable Meetings

Template reporting contributed to efficiently communicating what was happening, with an opportunity to focus on the unexpected. It enabled us to get through the financial presentation quickly because the template was identical at each meeting and all knew what each piece of information meant at each place on the template. The financial template covered the previous 5 fiscal years, the current year or part thereof, and a forecast for the next 3 fiscal years. We could quickly skim the data, ask about the anomalies and move on to the more important non-financial data. This was consistent with our operating philosophy that financial results are trailing consequences of what we do. Delivering fiscal results isn't what we do. We do things in pursuit of our vision to be the leader in improving child health. The financial results come from that, and while important, they aren't where we want to focus our attention. Our focus is on how we will be safer, more accessible, more patient engaged. Being able to understand financial results in the least time possible in our business unit meetings was substantially enhanced by use of template reporting.

Similarly we sought to report on safety, access and other initiatives through templates as much as possible. This was harder because there is no similarly developed accounting system for these areas. Still, having consistent, standardized reports accelerated our ability to discuss the important dimensions of what was happening, why, and what was needed to accelerate improvement.

Predictable, scheduled meetings with the business unit leaders and the medical center leaders are critical. Our business units initially met quarterly and then three times a year. In virtually every case, each of the three business unit leaders for each of the 15-plus business units was present at each meeting over many years. Similarly the CEO, chief financial officer (CFO), chief nursing officer, chief medical officer, chief information officer, chief quality officer, our leaders of human resources and strategic planning and business development, and other senior leaders (15 in total) were present for presentations in their area of responsibility. I missed only a few over a decade.

The compelling truth is that with predictable, recurring meetings with the most senior leadership of the business unit and the institution, there is no place to hide. If an issue of operational excellence is addressed at the May meeting and not resolved, all know that the fall meeting will provide another opportunity to discuss it, and progress will be expected. That is true whether the business unit owes the institutional leadership an answer, or whether the institution owes the business unit an answer. There is no escape from accountability – either way.

Predictable meetings permitted us to advance long-term goals like improved outcomes by disease. When we began that initiative there were many uncertainties: how to choose the diseases or conditions to improve, how to define best practices and desired outcomes, how to measure and monitor our performance, who would be accountable, and how we would report progress. The business unit structure gave us a means for addressing all these challenges. Through the business unit structure, we asked each unit to identify three important diseases or conditions, measurements for each, and a plan of action to improve outcomes, incorporating process improvements and the results of research. Through our business unit meeting discussions, we could assure family centeredness, safety, and resource adequacy and appropriateness. We could also agree on a plan of action and monitor progress at each meeting. In short, through the dynamic business unit engagement, we could lead the improvement of child health with the sure knowledge that it was actually happening and that we had the data to prove it. We also could train each other in the way we each thought about problems and could brainstorm possible solutions, applying the full intellectual and financial resources of the institution.

A New Focus on Quality Improvement

The professional development of neonatologist Uma Kotagal, MD, took a new direction in the mid-1990s that provided the institution with an energized, insistent, and effective leader for improved quality. Frustrated with the institution's inability to deliver improved results and with the full support of the institution, she enrolled in a degree program for a Master of Science in Epidemiology (Clinical Effectiveness) at the Harvard School of Public Health to acquire the tools essential to apply new knowledge to improvement. Returning to Cincinnati Children's in 1996 with energy and skills to methodically improve outcomes, she found a new CEO with a special interest in applying these skills in the institution. Having a respected, seasoned physician with the interest and skills to transform the delivery system proved to be pivotal in our journey. Increasingly we were drawn together in our aspiration for a markedly improved delivery system. We now had the expertise for change management in the system, a management structure (business units) that could stimulate change and a board chair who embraced transformation. We needed focus and a plan.

Our vision began the focus. The Institute of Medicine reports on the safety and quality of the American health-care system contributed the dimensions we sought: timely, efficient, safe, effective, patient centered and equitable care. Our strategic planning process led to more detailed direction. By 1999, led by Dr. Kotagal, we had built a core resource for data collection and analysis as well as the capacity to assess clinical effectiveness of the care we were providing. We could demonstrate through data that the care was inconsistent, often not based on known best practices and produced varied results. The importance of the capacity to collect and analyze data cannot be overstated. It was an early investment for us and was the instrument for change common to all of our improvements. Good data were critical to engage physicians in improvement work, and the ability to design and redesign studies and track outcomes were essential to convincing clinicians to change. In addition, quality data were the language used to communicate the results of our efforts with the board, our external audiences and internally. Data kept the zeal for change robust.

Importantly, we had success at the micro level in materially changing our practices, leading to demonstrably better outcomes, reduced consumption of resources and clearly better experience for families. Encouraged by our experience, institutional leadership, including the board of trustees, was eager to move down the path of further, more widespread transformation. The result was our 2001 strategic plan, the development of which included extensive engagement by the board, faculty, staff, and business representatives. Pivotal influences were Dr. Cotton's observation that we should focus on improving our systems, Dr. Kotagal's expertise in improvement, the early encouraging results we had achieved, and our board chairman Lee Carter's unwavering commitment to constant improvement. Also important was leadership's embrace of family-centered care after a group of trustees, organizational leaders and frontline staff attended the national meeting of the Institute for Family-Centered Care in 1998.

As we engaged in developing the strategic plan, it became clearer to each of us how dysfunctional our delivery system was, how huge the opportunity was before us, and that we knew how to fix it. From the viewpoint of a CEO hungry to make our vision a reality, the direction for leadership became clear. We just had to figure out how to do what was required.

Concurrently, Lee Carter and I were discussing whether the board and its committee structure were aligned to be helpful in our journey. Lee noted that we had a research committee led by a marvelously stimulating, revolutionary board member, Geoff Place, a retired senior research executive from Procter & Gamble. Geoff's leadership had been instrumental in improving the infrastructure of our growing research endeavor (since 2006 we have been the second-highest recipient of National Institutes of Health funding for pediatric research, behind Boston Children's), and he was a very supportive, boundary-less thinker about Cincinnati Children's role in improving child health globally. With the example of a vigorous research committee, Lee asked which committee applied similar energy to the quality of our patient care. There was none.

In 1998, Lee created the patient care committee of the board, appointed himself as chair and established a charter that directed the committee to provide oversight to the institution's initiatives to improve patient care. Considerable apprehension followed. Would the committee comprised of trustees, parents and community appointees intrude into business they knew little about? Would the result be a distraction to the clinicians as they pursued their important work? Who would tell Lee that he shouldn't do this?

Happily, none of our fears were realized. With Lee's enthusiasm and regular definition of the roles of each of us, the committee brought useful focus on our improvement projects and the connection between things going wrong and improvement. He created a supportive but ambitious tone for management and staff, and conveyed to the board the priority of safe patient care.

One of his predictable requests – still being made regularly – was to understand harm in terms of individual patients and not just as a rate per thousand or other convention that would insulate us emotionally from the fact that these are real kids who got hurt while we were responsible.

Having the committee and the benefit of its deep exploration into our improvement initiative gave Lee the opportunity to convey the many messages associated with our initiative – both good and bad – to the full board at every meeting. That he did this with deep concern for patients and families, and that as chair of the board he chose also to chair this committee, changed the board and staff priorities. Each committee and board meeting begins with a safety report reviewing any new serious safety events and the status of recent ones. No longer was there any ambiguity about the importance of patient welfare in our institution. It was our first priority. We were structured to focus on it, and we did.

Energizing the Staff to Participate

Committed as the board and senior management were to transformation, the challenge became how to persuade the rest of the organization to think and act in a boundary-less fashion in pursuit of radically better outcomes and operations. My early efforts were to make the case – compelling to me – that success would bring greater efficiency, effectiveness and benefit to the community, especially the kids that we served.

All agreed. We knew we were on an unsustainable path of increasing cost, and that improvements to become more cost-effective were needed. No one pushed back that they were not persuaded. And no one changed his behavior. We had widespread efforts to persuade from the top, widespread agreement from the middle, and widespread business as usual.

Clearly we were missing something critical to energizing our very talented community to deliver change. After considerable thought and discussion, we concluded that while we had appealed to the logical minds of our staff, we had not spoken to their soul – to the fundamental, not always logical reasons they had committed to a career in health care in the first place. Our answer was to stop talking about money and focus solely on taking better care of kids. We bet that if we got the part right about taking better care of kids, the money would take care of itself. It couldn't be proved. It wasn't logical. It was risky, but we thought it would work. We made it clear that we would invest to enable any change in how we cared for kids that improved outcomes, without regard to the financial consequences. Clinicians should stop wondering about whether the institution really wanted to do that extra test, admit one more patient, or nurse one more infected patient back to health by keeping them in the hospital another three or four days. The answer became: "If it is good for child health, do it. If you need resources, you will get them. You deliver improved child health. We will worry about the money."

Skepticism and curiosity followed, then testing, then embrace, and finally zeal from the increasing freedom to follow the hopes they embraced when they first committed to a career in health care. We had connected to their deep motivation. That the institution would do this shouldn't have been a complete surprise. Several years earlier, under the leadership of Dr. Kotagal, the institution had developed protocols related to care of kids with asthma, bronchiolitis and fever of uncertain source, resulting in a reduction in admissions of kids with those conditions of between 20% and 50%. These were conditions that produced more admissions than any other, yet we invested resources to reduce them. The literature supported our protocols – indeed they were derived from the literature, but their adoption was slow at the outset. Nevertheless what we did reflected institutional support for radical change to take better care of kids even at the expense of reduced revenue.

An incident several years after we changed how we communicated our quality initiative reflects how hard it was to convince everyone that we meant what we said. In 2002, Dr. Kotagal began a seminar called Intermediate Improvement Science Seminar, I^2S^2 for short. Its purpose was to equip middle- to upper-level managers with deep knowledge about the process of change and how to lead it, an explicit recognition of the importance of professional development if the gains in outcome and system performance were to be realized and sustained. Each participant was required to do an improvement project. Students met 2 full days a month offsite for 6 months. Participants included division directors, unit nurses, senior managers, business directors and others who were essential to widespread change. To demonstrate the institutional commitment to improvement, our board chair, CEO, and CFO each spoke, stressing the critical importance of quality improvement to our organization. At one such meeting, after the CFO spoke, a physician director asked how we would react to disruptive change that had significant benefits for kids but would reduce the institution's revenue. Scott Hamlin, our CFO and a tireless advocate for our change strategy, assured the physician that we were truly interested in such improvements, that she should bring the proposal to him and that we would be glad to help her get it done. I jumped up to interrupt and said, "Just do it. If it is good for kids, we want you to make the changes. We don't want to create barriers to those changes. You take better care of kids. Scott and I will worry about the finances."

The I^2S^2 sessions were rich opportunities to advance the professional development of hundreds of clinicians and business leaders. Participants learned techniques, read the literature, led their own improvement projects, and learned convincingly the institution's commitment to improvement, transparency, and providing leadership in improving child health. As learners became proficient leaders of change, they knew of the resources offered to support their continuing search for opportunities to improve care for kids. They knew how to apply improvement science techniques. Through Dr. Kotagal's department, they had access to experts in data collection and analysis, lean techniques, Six Sigma, and the PDSA (Plan-Do-Study-Act) improvement process to support their work over the long term.

We wanted to create the motivation for change in the divisions and then make it easy to execute. We wanted improvement to be part of the everyday work of each division. We wanted leaders to know the institution would support their boldest efforts. I^2S^2 sessions gave us a chance to reinforce how interdependent we all are, how we are all in this together and how each of us has an obligation to the other to make excellence habitual. The opportunity to do this is why we are all together, and only together will we be able to make the contribution to improved child health that is our promise.

Pursuing Perfection

Soon after the board approved our 2001 strategic plan, the Robert Wood Johnson Foundation announced an initiative titled "Pursuing Perfection: Raising the Bar for Healthcare Performance," to be administered by the Institute for Healthcare Improvement (IHI) headed by Don Berwick. A grant of more than $2 million over 2 years was available to a few model institutions that the IHI judged to be ready, willing and able to make transformational change in pursuit of perfection. They sought to encourage exactly the behavior we had committed to in our strategic plan. The thought of being contractually committed to Robert Wood Johnson Foundation, be paid for our efforts and most importantly be hardwired through IHI into the best thinking about radical change was irresistible. Following several site visits of increasing rigor, in which 100 or more of us participated, we became one of the seven participants.

A requirement that came with the grant that gave us all some pause was a commitment to transparency. The grant advanced our thinking about transparency and unleashed an enormously helpful force for change within the institution. We came to share good and bad results with patients and families, to post data on numerous conditions – surgical site infections, mortality rates, ventilator associated pneumonia and many others – on our website, and to post prominently on our intranet home page the number of days since the last serious safety event, as well as days since the last employee lost time injury. We told parents of patients with cystic fibrosis that we were not getting nearly the good results of other centers, and if they wanted to move the care of their child to another higher performing center we would help them. We met with parents of children injured at Cincinnati Children's within hours or minutes of an adverse event. We told them all that we knew and followed up as we learned more. We took responsibility, helped them find lawyers and committed to fixing the system so the same thing didn't happen to another child.

Each of these practices was painful but essential to exhibit without reservation our highest commitment to taking better care of kids. The message communicated by our transparency was most important to our internal audience. It said more clearly than words could that taking care of kids was our highest priority. No ambiguity; no winking; no public message different from private behavior.

Insistence on excellence didn't always deliver excellence. Kids still got hurt, some died because we didn't perform to potential. With transparency, we all knew of more incidents of harm and near misses than before. Atul Gwande, MD, wrote in the *New Yorker*[3] about how we discovered that our outcomes on critical measures for cystic fibrosis patients were at the 20th percentile. Crushing, painful news widely spread yet it was fair commentary; the facts were accurate and they were delivered with such clarity that caring people could do nothing but commit to improvement or perpetual embarrassment. The unavoidable message was that we can do better and out of these increasingly visible, disappointing experiences came increased determination to eliminate them by improving what we delivered.

A New Mission Statement

Within a few years we were ready to produce a new strategic plan. We had had success with our improvement agenda and were ready to push the frontiers further. After nine months of numerous groups working separately to develop our objectives, a team of trustees, physician and nurse leadership and senior management came together to integrate our initiatives. In doing that we affirmed our vision – to be the leader in improving child health – but rejected our mission statement, which had been written in 1986. It was nothing more than a wordy inventory of what we did. It had no energy, no direction and no inspiration. In two weeks we wrote another:

Cincinnati Children's will improve child health and transform delivery of care through fully integrated, globally recognized research, education and innovation.

For patients from our community, the nation and the world, the care we provide will achieve the best
- medical and quality of life outcomes

- patient and family experience
- value.

Today and in the future.

Our new mission statement committed us to improvement, to integration, to research and to innovation. Importantly it said we would deliver improved outcomes, experience and value, each measurable, over the long term. The most revolutionary phrase in it is "fully integrated," an idea offered by a physician faculty member. The notion of thinking of our potential as derived from the application of fully integrated institutional resources was a breakthrough. It said we would accept no silos – no separation of outcomes, system performance, and professional development. It recognized the interdependence of each and the requirement of habitual excellence from each. The three components aren't a triangle, each corner connected but developing in relative isolation; they are intertwined components on a flywheel, each adding strength, enlightenment and energy to the other and together contributing to the speed and energy of the flywheel.[4]

As I reflect on the relationship among the triangle of patient outcomes, operational excellence, and professional development through the filter of my experience at Cincinnati Children's, I am increasingly of the view that integrated management is essential to achieve excellence throughout. To the extent any point on the triangle is left to develop without hard-wired connections and assured interaction with the others, potential is lost. An implication of this conclusion is that integrated medical centers need to take greater responsibility for the perfection of our health-care system and each of its components. At these institutions, and only these, is there the opportunity – and I would argue, the duty – to integrate outcomes, operations and development of professionals, to apply the learning of each to the other and pursue habitual excellence across the complex spectrum of interests that is our health-care system. These institutions are the commons, and out of effective use of the commons will come improved health.

My hope is that this narrative will prove provocative and useful. Let me conclude by summarizing eight key messages:

1. All the points of the triangle – patient outcomes, operational excellence and professional development – have to perform well for any to perform to potential.
2. To perform well, an institution needs a shared, compelling vision, an energetic mission, a strategic plan informed by data but not data driven, and action plans characterized by accountability and transparency.
3. Mechanisms to deliver the vision, mission, strategic plan, and action plan

    must be hard-wired and predictable, and must foster agility (i.e., business units).

4. A single hierarchy with obligations to serve and accountability for results on all points of the triangle is desirable.

5. One should institutionalize thinking without boundaries, risk taking, transparency, small tests of change (not business as usual).

6. Set high expectations for everyone.

7. Organizational structure reflects priorities. There won't be transformational change without transformed structure.

8. Base the organization's vision, mission, strategic plans, and actions on the values that draw people to health care. The job of leaders is to enable fellow believers to deliver their best, to create an environment where all have justified, absolute faith in the institutional commitment to delivering the best. Then do it.

I want to thank Beatrice Katz, PhD, Senior Associate, Marketing and Communications, Cincinnati Children's Hospital Medical Center, for her invaluable editorial assistance.

References

1. Kohn LT, Corrigan JM, Donaldson MS, editors. *To Err is Human: building a safer health system.* Washington, DC: National Academies Press; 1999.

2. Committee on Quality of Health Care in America, Institute of Medicine. *Crossing the Quality Chasm: a new health system for the 21st century.* Washington, DC: National Academies Press; 2001.

3. Gwande A. The bell curve. *New Yorker.* December 6, 2004.

4. Collins J. *Good to Great: why some companies make the leap … and others don't.* New York, NY: Harper Business; 2001.

9

The Triangle and Undergraduate Medical Education

Jonathan Huntington, Linda Headrick, and Greg Ogrinc

Introduction

John Allen has been a pulmonologist and inpatient medicine attending physician at Parkview Academic Medical Center for over 30 years. He came north to Parkview in 1977 after completing medical school in the south. He never envisioned that he'd enjoy the northern clime, but it's been a good career for him at Parkview. Lately, he's been frustrated by the increased demands that accompany clinical teaching: duty hour restrictions on resident physicians, new competencles about systems and improvement, and medical students who seem better able than he to find and integrate the latest medical evidence. It seemed so simple in the past ... patients were admitted to the hospital and stayed as long as they needed, so students and residents had plenty of time for a deep understanding of each patient's medical issues. Now there are administrators – some even with medical degrees – who monitor length of stay and clinical processes. The revolving door on the inpatient service is challenging for him. Dr. Allen recognizes that these are important matters, but they get in the way of teaching and delivering care. Some days it just feels like these new demands are like trying to fit a square peg in a round hole.

While the content of undergraduate medical education (UME) has been changing at an exponential rate in the 100 years since Abraham Flexner published his seminal report *Medical Education in the United States and Canada* in 1910,[1] much of the basic framework in which this education is delivered has remained the same. Medical students arrive at the start of medical school with basic knowledge in the biological, chemical, and physical sciences. Over the next 4 years they embark on a journey in professional development that is remarkably similar to that of students who entered the profession several generations ago. However, much has changed within this time span: tremendous societal transformation; an explosion in the amount, accessibility, and depth of scientific knowledge; and broad shifts in how we finance and deliver health care.[2] As highlighted in the vignette, these changing dynamics pose significant challenges to the current medical education system and have many medical educators looking for innovative ways to educate future generations of physicians.

How Can the Triangle Diagram Help?

The current prevailing structure of UME is built on a model where "preclinical" and "clinical" education are temporally separated. The former takes the form of classroom-based instruction and discussion of normal physiology, pathophysiology, and the scientific basis of disease-specific therapy. Armed with this foundation, medical students are sent out to clinical settings in the latter years of their training in order to gain firsthand experience in the application of the knowledge and skills which they have begun to develop during these early "preclinical" years. This educational pathway is primarily focused on only one domain articulated in the triangle diagram – "professional development." Students are expected to concentrate primarily on developing their own learning – much of this is focused in a disease or skill-specific manner filtered through the care of individual patients. The implicit (and sometimes explicit) structure of our current educational system asserts that if we prepare students properly by cultivating learner-specific knowledge, skills, and attitudes, they can be placed within a health care delivery system in an apprentice role and through a process of legitimate peripheral participation,[3] can continue to develop those skills to the point where they achieve competency sufficient to improve outcomes one patient at a time. This process is linear, beginning with the input of "professional development" and ending with an expected outcome of "better patient outcomes." However, there is little to no preparation of students in the skills and knowledge needed to understand and impact "system performance," with much of this domain being relegated to the form of a "mist" in the background of their experiences, obscured from the learner and clinicians (*see* Figure 9.1). Knowledge and thinking about the performance of the system of care delivery is separated from the professional development of students, resident physicians, or attending physicians.

Furthermore, different professionals tend each domain, potentially segregating them into separate silos. System performance is the purview of administrators, professional development is in the hands of education leaders, and frontline

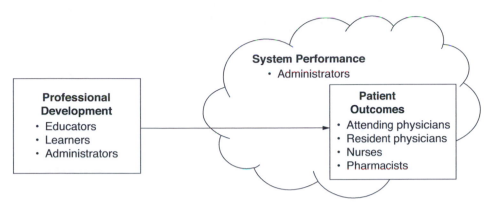

FIGURE 9.1 "Deconstructed" triangle diagram

clinicians are responsible for better patient outcomes. This delineation of domains and responsibilities makes some intuitive sense but also creates professional silos and fractures systems that are, in reality, enmeshed. To complicate matters further, learners are seldom educated as to what constitutes a better outcome on both an individual patient level and a population level. The end result of such a linear, deconstructed model is an educational experience that is fragmented and often leaves learners feeling bewildered and frustrated by their seeming inability to affect "the system."

The triangle diagram breaks this linearity and explicitly recognizes that care is delivered within a system. It advocates for simultaneous attention to each domain – arguing that since each is inextricably linked, educators must prepare students to be competent in all domains, no longer accepting the assumption that care will be improved simply by focusing on an individual's professional development (in the form of medical knowledge and patient care). Developing competence begins with the recognition that each domain is equally important, but also requires that medical students have meaningful experiential learning opportunities in systems that value each domain. The triangle diagram also integrates patients and families as co-designers of care and confronts much of what we currently deliver as a part of the "hidden curriculum" – those unintended teachings not found in the formal curriculum but made explicit by our actions.[4] While we are not aware that such a fully integrated system exists currently, many have recognized the limitations of our current educational system and have begun to construct curricula that are consistent with the multiple domains articulated in the triangle diagram.[5]

An Exemplary Care and Learning Site
· ·

Learning cannot be separated from the context in which it is delivered. If we want medical students to embrace all domains of the triangle, we must provide them meaningful experiential learning opportunities in a system where this is the norm. What would such a site look like? How would it function?

One model is the exemplary care and learning site (ECLS). An ECLS is "a clinical care site that produces patient-centered care in a way that continually improves patient outcomes, system performance, and professional development."[6] The ECLS model builds from the foundation of the triangle, which sits at its center (*see* Figure 9.2) and identifies five elements necessary to translate the theory articulated by the triangle into daily practice. At such a site, there is explicit integration of teaching by clinicians and leaders who are actively engaged in not only delivering high-quality care, but also using the learning afforded by continuous quality improvement to improve care at both the individual patient and population levels. Learners in an ECLS see these processes modeled by their teachers. They can learn in depth how all the elements of the system come together to ensure that patients receive care that is effective, timely, safe and responsive to their needs. Creation of an ECLS requires leadership around a shared vision that draws from all the players within the delivery system.

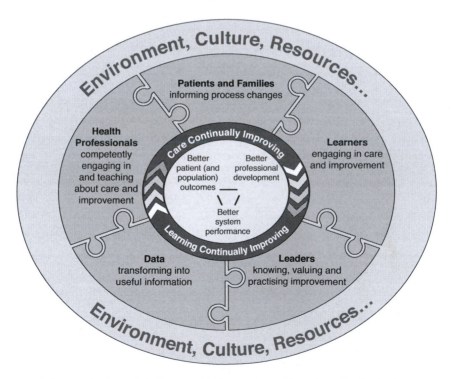

FIGURE 9.2 Conceptual model of an exemplary care and learning site (ECLS)

The Five Elements of an Exemplary Care and Learning Site as it Relates to Undergraduate Medical Education

An ECLS values and embraces the education of learners at all levels and in all professions. Below we discuss each of the five elements of an ECLS, paying particular attention to how it relates to undergraduate medical education. We will follow with examples of ECLS from specific sites. While our discussion is focused on undergraduate medical education, one can apply the concepts to learners at all stages and from all health care professions.

Leaders

Leaders in the ECLS know the power of applying the science of improvement to health care delivery. They understand that care is delivered within a system and use quality improvement (QI) in their daily work. This serves as a model to others, and makes it explicit that they value improvement. Specifically, ECLS leaders know what resources are needed to provide quality care and education and what tools are needed to work to improve each on a continuous basis (data, time, space, personnel, and so forth). Finally, an ECLS recognizes that effective leadership is seldom provided by a single individual and instead is shared by all members of an interprofessional team.

Patients

An ECLS seeks out patients and families as active partners in informing process changes. The degree of patient and family partnership can fall along a wide spectrum, ranging from an individual patient's active involvement in his or her own care to the development of advisory boards, all the way to a full partnership with patients and families in the improvement and co-design of systems and processes of care.[7] Advisory boards are one example of organization units in which the voice of patients and families can be usefully and actively integrated into processes that drive the design and improvement of care. Examples include program development, implementation and evaluation; design of a new building or service; and staff selection and training. Partnership with patients and families requires ECLS leaders to work at selecting, activating and educating patients and families in a manner similar to what we do to recruit and prepare other members of improvement teams.

Health Professionals

Health professionals in the ECLS must be competent in the knowledge and skills of improvement. In order for this to occur, all health professionals must have firsthand experience in improvement, incorporating it into their daily work. This intimate knowledge and integration into daily practice allows for the modeling and teaching necessary within the ECLS. This serves both the patients and families currently receiving care within the ECLS and the future patients who will be served by the health professionals being trained there.

The ECLS, with its focus on the system of care, recognizes the interprofessional nature of health care delivery and highlights that there are many professionals who work together to deliver care. This list is not just limited to clinicians but also includes ward clerks, unit secretaries and other staff members. Each of these individuals contributes to the education of learners within the ECLS. The end result is that this educational process does not occur in discrete episodes separated from daily work, but is built into the regular patterns of the care delivery system.

Learners

Medical student learners are required to develop competence in providing care. They also need to learn to assess and improve the system within which they work. The best improvement education incorporates both didactics and meaningful experiential learning with students serving as an active part of the improvement team. In doing so, the ECLS provides an opportunity for learners to practice and reflect in a way that integrates these experiences with the foundational knowledge about systems that they are simultaneously receiving. Often learners benefit greatly from coaching as they negotiate the difficulties of learning to both provide and improve care. This model of education is hardwired into the ECLS and thus serves as required core content. It is not an elective learning experience or just reserved for potential future leaders. The ECLS recognizes that all learners benefit from this education.

Data

Data serve an important role within an ECLS as the only "nonhuman" element. Data within the ECLS must be visible, actionable, timely, balanced, easily available, publically displayed, and provide insight into the functioning of the system. These data are utilized to directly inform improvement work and guide the process of exerting action on the system. Simply put, feedback is the fuel of learning and data provide that feedback. Data for improvement are often different from data for research or for accountability.[8] While an ECLS may utilize each of these types of data, data for improvement hold a special place within the ECLS, guiding and shaping changes in daily work.

The Exemplary Care and Learning Site as an Integrated Model

While the five elements highlighted are the foundation of the ECLS model, none functions in isolation from the whole. The model arranges the elements in dynamic and interlocking relationships with one another around the triangle diagram at its center. These elements and relationships are embedded in the surrounding mantle of the local context (environment, culture, resources, and so forth). Explicit in this model is the recognition that the force that holds each of these elements in relationship is the "Everyone" at the core of the triangle. In other words, in order for the ECLS to reach its fullest potential, each stakeholder (patient, leader, clinician, learner, staff, and so forth) must work in partnership to optimize the ideal outcomes (system performance, outcomes, professional development) articulated by the triangle.

Does an Exemplary Care and Learning Site Exist Currently?

Now that we have highlighted the ideal objectives of the ECLS model, let's ask an important question – does such a site exist currently? Do students participate as full partners within any current system? The following section describes specific examples where medical students have been engaged as learners at sites striving to reach the potential embodied in both the ECLS model and the triangle diagram. We examine each of these through the lens of the ECLS model, using each of the five elements described as a framework to highlight where progress has been made and where opportunities for improvement exist.

Dartmouth Medical School

Since 2006, Dartmouth Medical School has offered an elective rotation for second-year medical students called the Health Leadership Practicum (HeLP).[9] The goal of this elective is for students to apply the knowledge and skills of QI to a project. Initially, students worked on nonclinical projects such as evaluating the student mentoring system at the medical school. While this was a reasonable starting point, it lacked any connection to clinical care and patient outcomes. It allowed students to gain some experience with QI tools, but to make the elective experience more meaningful, the work needed to be connected to clinical sites.

Clinical sites were chosen based on key components of the ECLS model: leaders who support QI work, clinicians who are engaged in QI work, and readily available data. While none of the sites could be described as a fully functional ECLS site, careful attention to these characteristics has made the experience successful for students and faculty. One site is at Alice Peck Day Hospital – a small, rural community hospital located close to Dartmouth Medical School. The director of the obstetrics and gynecology clinic, Susan Mooney, MD, MS, is a graduate of the Veterans Administration Quality Scholars Fellowship Program.[10] Dr. Mooney has knowledge, skills, and passion for improving the effectiveness and efficiency of care for the patients in the obstetrics and gynecology clinic. She led the development of a clinical site that regularly uses data to evaluate

TABLE 9.1 Curricular Programs that Demonstrate One or More of the Exemplary Care and Learning Site Elements

Institution	Leaders Knowing, Valuing and Practicing Improvement	Patients and Families Informing Process Changes	Health Professionals Engage in and Teach about Improvement	Learners Engaging in Care and Improvement	Data Transforming into Useful Information
Dartmouth Medical School	Sites are chosen that have leaders who are ready to support improvement	No	Not explicitly, but improvement has been intermittently part of each site	Learners are present to improve the system, not to deliver care	Yes, data must be available for learners to participate
University of Missouri-Columbia	Strong connection of student work on reducing falls to important organizational initiatives	No	Faculty involved in the teaching of delivery of care and improvement of care	Medical and nursing students evaluating and making changes to reduce patient falls during their clinical rotations delivering care	Yes, patient falls data are key in the feedback loop to student work
Colorado Children's Hospital	Educational leader and chief quality officer collaborate for the curriculum	No	Nursing students work directly with nursing faculty on improved communication; fewer opportunities for medical students	Students focus on collecting data about standard communication; this occurs as part of usual educational rotations	Yes, students engaged in collecting data that are meaningful to action

the clinical care and has started developing the professional staff to contribute to continuous improvement. She has hosted several HeLP student groups over the past several years. Student work has led to increased influenza vaccine rate for expectant mothers and to increased prenatal urine testing. The success of the QI projects at Alice Peck Day is directly related to Dr. Mooney's leadership, which has instilled a culture of improvement for staff and is guided by the availability of data.

For the episodic student improvement work that comes with an elective rotation, this site functions exceptionally well; however to take full advantage of the ECLS model, two elements would need to be strengthened. First, the frontline staff would need to be actively and continually engaged in QI. Perhaps having learners present all the time and always engaged in QI would be a motivating factor for the clinical setting. The students and the staff would be co-learners in the development of effective and efficient care.[11] Second, the site would benefit from patient involvement in the QI work. For example, patients were not involved in the influenza vaccine project, but an understanding of barriers to receiving the vaccine – directly from patient participation on the QI team – might enhance the development of effective interventions.

The Dartmouth HeLP elective has spread beyond Alice Peck Day hospital to community primary care clinics, the White River Junction Veterans Affairs Hospital, and Dartmouth-Hitchcock Medical Center. The learning from the initial work at Alice Peck Day has provided guidelines for success at these other sites. Each project by students is lead by a site coach with knowledge and skills in QI and readily available data. These are now written requirements for sites that want to have a student team. The penetration of QI to frontline staff is variable at each site, but all are welcoming of students engaging in improvement activity. While this remains an elective, episodic activity and considerable work must be done to create the reliable and stable ECLS where students (and all learners) participate in improvement as the routine part of care delivery, this experience serves as a model and is helping to guide ongoing curriculum reform efforts at Dartmouth.

University of Missouri School of Medicine

The University of Missouri Schools of Medicine and Nursing (in Columbia, Missouri) established The Integrated Interprofessional Patient Safety (TIIPS) curriculum in 2009 as part of the Institute for Healthcare Improvement's "Retooling for Quality and Safety" initiative, with support from the Josiah Macy Jr. Foundation.[12] The interprofessional faculty team uses fall prevention as a way to integrate patient safety into the core curriculum of each school: the Internal Medicine Year 3 clerkship for medical students and a required medical-surgical clinical course for nursing students. For the School of Medicine, this experience builds on prior quality improvement and patient safety curricula that occur in the classroom and the simulation center in years one and two.[13]

The experience includes four components: (1) independent study on patient safety, quality improvement, and fall risk reduction; (2) an interprofessional simulation experience in which students adopt handicaps (like vision-distorting glasses and intravenous lines) to learn about preventing falls in older adults; (3) pairs of medical and nursing students performing an inpatient bedside fall risk on one of their patients to design a customized fall reduction patient education plan; and (4) a small group interprofessional debriefing conference to consolidate learning about core principles of patient safety, basic methods of effective interprofessional teamwork, and a systems-approach to patient safety and quality improvement.

The TIIPS curriculum takes advantage of three ECLS elements present at University of Missouri Health Care's (MU Health Care's) medical inpatient units: (1) leaders who know, value, and practice improvement; (2) health professionals engaging in and teaching improvement; and (3) data that is regularly transformed into useful information. MU Health Care leaders have invested in quality improvement since the mid-1990s, an effort recently recognized with the 2011 Missouri Quality Award. TIIPS students' work on falls prevention contributes to the institution's fall prevention activities. In this context the faculty identified a specific meaningful task for student teams (patient-specific fall reduction plans) and built a learning experience that includes preparation (pre-readings), action (bedside fall risk assessment), and reflection (small group discussion).

Missing from the experience is "patients/families informing process changes." MU Health Care has an active Patient and Family Advisory Council that meets monthly and provides input to a variety of health system initiatives. Patient and family member volunteers served as members of the team that planned the move of pediatric inpatient services to the new Women's and Children's Hospital.[14] Although patients and families are infrequently part of clinical improvement efforts that also involve students, both patient and student representatives actively participate in the University of Missouri School of Medicine's "Next Level of Excellence" Steering Committee for medical student education. Expanding opportunities for medical students to work in partnership with patients to improve care would add a new dimension to students' understanding of effective quality improvement.

Children's Hospital Colorado

Matt Vitaska, ND, RN, at Children's Hospital Colorado (CHC) has developed an interprofessional curriculum for nursing and medical students to learn the basic foundation of quality improvement and apply this learning during clinical rotations. Each month, about 25 nursing students and four medical students work together in the QI rotation. Dr. Vitaska begins with students using the Institute for Healthcare Improvement Open School (www.IHI.org) online modules. Students review these as a way to build basic knowledge about core principles. This is combined with videos, discussions, and explicit links to CHC organizational efforts about QI and safety, which sets the stage for students to understand the local issues and the organizational factors involved in the QI work. Students work to apply this foundational knowledge through participation in two QI projects.

First, students work on reducing patient misidentification events, making sure the right patient is identified for the right procedure at the right time. While the staff has regular QI meetings about this work, students participate in those sporadically. Students collect data about the patient identification proc-ess and the ongoing QI work, thus providing vital feedback to the QI team that is not available through other data sources. Second, students assist with the evaluation of handoffs on the unit. These include provider-to-provider as well as unit-to-unit handoffs. After learning about and practicing standard handoff and communication techniques such as SBAR (Situation, Background, Assessment, Recommendation), the students observe and collect data about the fidelity of handoffs on the unit. Students have improved the data collection tools, provided process measure data such as staff satisfaction, used a structured data format, and monitored outcomes such as care failures. These data were not available from other sources, so they provided a more complete assessment for the site about its improvement work. At the end of the rotation, the students reflect upon their experience in a small group session.

The CHC work provides a good example of how a site combines the learning about improvement (through online and classroom activities) and the doing of improvement on a clinical unit. Because the usual data sources are not adequate, the students act as observers and data gatherers in this system, thus learning an important point about ensuring that data are at the proper level to take action. While the CHC students do not have direct patient or family involvement in their ECLS, there is strong support from educational and care delivery leaders. This is combined with the active QI work of staff and faculty, a process that provides important modeling for the students.

The Role of Patients and Families

In each of the examples given, educators have worked to combine different ECLS elements as a means to reach the desired outcomes articulated by the triangle diagram of better patient outcomes, better professional development and better system performance. Each site has done this in a slightly different way. None to date have put together all the elements, but all have made progress. The most obvious domain where these sites have yet to fully engage is the area of patient and family involvement. This is perhaps not surprising given the difficulty of bridging the substantial gap between embracing the concept and actually practicing "patient-centered care" in daily work. Redesigning health care processes from the patient's perspective remains a significant goal of many current improvement efforts, where a direct partnership with the end users can be beneficial. Paul Bate and Glen Robert[15] articulated such a model of co-design and argued that the value in incorporating knowledge from patients' previous experiences into the design or improvement of systems leads directly to better future patient experiences. This places the experience goals of patients and families at the center of the design and improvement process and assigns it equal value to process efficiency and clinical goals. As more health care organizations develop and embrace models of active partnership with patient family advisors and advisory councils, patients and family members will play increasingly important roles in both the work of improving current systems of care and the education of health professionals in improvement science.

The Exemplary Care and Learning Site: Getting Started
• •

While the ECLS model conceptualizes one method to operationalize and realize the outcomes articulated by the triangle diagram, a fully functional ECLS does not need to be in place before substantive work can begin. On the contrary, as evidenced by the case examples above, not all elements of the ECLS need be fully present before health professionals, leaders, learners, and patients can begin to reap the benefits of a more integrated system of care delivery and professional development. Furthermore, Cooke *et al.*[11] argue that health professional students and their clinical teachers must become co-learners while working together to improve patient outcomes and systems of care. The improvement of care cannot wait for teachers to build expertise, but rather teachers and learners can and should build competence together.

TABLE 9.2 Tips for Recognizing the Degree to which the Exemplary Care and Learning Site (ECLS) Elements are Present in a Potential ECLS site

ECLS Element	Getting Started	Intermediate	Advanced
Leaders	Leaders passively allow health professionals to engage in and teach about improvement	Leaders encourage others to lead and teach about improvement but model and support these practices inconsistently	Leaders model, expect and support continuous improvement consistently as a part of their daily work
In-career health professionals	One faculty member with experience in quality improvement who serves as a local champion	Core group of faculty who engage in, continuously learn, and teach about improvement intermittently while providing clinical care	All health professionals are continuously engaged in and teaching and learning about improvement as a part of their daily work
Learners (students and graduate trainees)	Learners work to identify and describe gaps between local and best practice in order to propose potential improvements	Learners identify gaps and work to pilot proposed improvements under the guidance of a mentor or coach	Learners are fully integrated into the improvement process serving as equal partners on improvement teams
Patients and families	Patients are engaged in their own care	Patients and families serve as advisors in focus groups or advisory councils	Patients and family members are equal partners on improvement teams
Data (information guiding learning)	Chart review to extract salient data on a small group of select patients	Ad hoc data query on a larger cohort of patients within the population of interest	Data automatically extracted, analyzed, and fed back to team in real time to guide improvement

In Table 9.2 we have tabulated representative examples of what might be found across the full spectrum within each ECLS element, from what it might look like at a site just starting out, to one that is further along in the ECLS developmental journey. We hope that this table will both provide a framework to evaluate the current strengths and weaknesses at a site and give a sense of places one might develop further while working towards becoming a fully functioning ECLS.

It may be helpful to illustrate how this matrix can be perspective-setting. Consider the "Data" row in the matrix. Currently, not all clinical sites have robust data extraction systems that can deliver actionable, real-time feedback to guide improvement. However, much can be learned by gathering and analyzing data from a small cohort of patients. Students could either work to collect these data themselves – such as in the case of Children's Hospital Colorado – or be steered towards units where these data have already been collected as was the case in the Dartmouth example. Similarly, while strong support from and engagement of leaders is vital to advancing the work of an ECLS, many improvements can still be achieved at sites where leaders provide only passive support, but do not impede the work. In either case the important first step is to begin the work with whatever resources are present or can be readily arranged. Once the improvement work has been initiated, further progress along the spectrum in each ECLS element can be targeted (e.g., building more robust data extraction systems or cultivating more active leadership engagement). Similar recommendations for each ECLS element are provided in Table 9.2.

Conclusion

Recently, Dr. Allen noticed that care seems to be a bit different on ward 1-South. One of the junior hospitalists has started to work with students (medical and nursing) and resident physicians to improve the discharge process for the patients and families. The student teams, working with the unit secretary, post charts of the percentage of discharges before noon each day. Dr. Allen also saw students testing a discharge checklist for the unit staff and for patients and families ... hmm ... interesting ... activating patients and families as partners in the discharge process. What has impressed him most about watching these activities is that they don't seem to take away from patient care. To his observation, the students are *more* engaged in patient care now than they had been in the past. Perhaps all these new demands and pressures on health care delivery can be resolved in conjunction with students as they learn to navigate and improve systems?

Historically, undergraduate medical education has focused almost entirely on the singular domain of professional development, believing that if learners are given enough medical knowledge and patient care skills, they will be able to successfully bring about improvements in patient outcomes. This model has been blind to the system in which care is delivered, and has supported the development of silos where clinicians, educators, and administrators often work in isolation. The triangle diagram describes the explicit interrelatedness of the desired goals of any improvement activity and broadens the gaze beyond a narrow construct of professional development. The ECLS model provides a framework for operationalizing the vision articulated by the triangle diagram. It outlines key elements that when put in place can lead to both improved care delivery and health professional education. Several academic medical centers have begun to build sites that embrace multiple ECLS elements and provide valuable educational experiences to students. Considerable work is needed to fully realize the promise of a true ECLS, particularly the element of partnering with patient and families, but ample opportunities exist. The ideals embraced by the ECLS model can bring about global improvements in patient outcomes, system performance and professional development.

Acknowledgment

The authors wish to thank Dr. Wendy Madigosky from the University of Colorado for her assistance with the preparation of this chapter.

References

1. Cooke M, Irby DM, O'Brien BC. *Educating physicians: a call for reform of medical school and residency.* 1st ed. San Francisco, CA: Jossey-Bass; 2010.
2. Starr P. *The Social Transformation of American Medicine.* New York, NY: Basic Books; 1982.
3. Lave J, Wenger E. *Situated Learning: legitimate peripheral participation.* Cambridge: Cambridge University Press; 1991.
4. Hafferty FW. Beyond curriculum reform: confronting medicine's hidden curriculum. *Acad Med.* 1998; **73**(4): 403–7.
5. Irby DM, Cooke M, O'Brien BC. Calls for reform of medical education by the Carnegie Foundation for the Advancement of Teaching: 1910 and 2010. *Acad Med.* 2010; **85**(2): 220–7.
6. Headrick LA, Shalaby M, Baum KD, *et al.* Exemplary care and learning sites: linking the continual improvement of learning and the continual improvement of care. *Acad Med.* 2011; **86**(11): e6–7.
7. Bate P, Robert G. Experience-based design: from redesigning the system around the patient to co-designing services with the patient. *Qual Saf Health Care.* 2006; **15**(5): 307–10.
8. Ogrinc G, Headrick L, editors. *Fundamentals of Health Care Improvement.* 2nd ed. Oakbrook Terrace, IL: Joint Commission Resources; 2012.
9. Ogrinc G, Nierenberg DW, Batalden PB. Building experiential learning about quality improvement into a medical school curriculum: the Dartmouth experience. *Health Aff (Millwood).* 2011; **30**(4): 716–22.
10. Splaine ME, Ogrinc G, Gilman SC, *et al.* The Department of Veterans Affairs National

Quality Scholars Fellowship Program: experience from 10 years of training quality scholars. *Acad Med.* 2009; **84**(12): 1741–8.

11. Cooke M, Ironside PM, Ogrinc GS. Mainstreaming quality and safety: a reformulation of quality and safety education for health professions students. *BMJ Qual Saf.* 2011; **20**(Suppl. 1): i79–82.

12. Dyer C, Gregory G, Aud M, *et al.* Using fall prevention for interprofessional patient safety training at the bedside. *Presented at Academy for Healthcare Improvement Scientific Symposium.* Orlando, FL; 2010.

13. Headrick LA, Hoffman KG, Brown RM, *et al.* University of Missouri School of Medicine in Columbia. *Acad Med.* 2010; **85**(9 Suppl.): S310–15.

14. Smith D. An academic medical center's journey toward teaching and delivering patient-centered care. In: Headrick LA and Litzelman DK, editors. *Enhancing the Professional Culture of Academic Health Science Centers: the interplay among education leaders, their programs, and the organizational environment.* London: Radcliffe Publishing; In Press.

15. Bate P, Robert G. *Bringing User Experience to Healthcare Improvement: the concepts, methods and practices of experience-based design.* Oxford: Radcliffe Publishing; 2007.

10

Triangle Synergies in a National Quality and Safety Education Initiative in Nursing

Linda R. Cronenwett and Pamela M. Ironside

The Patient Safety Advisory Committee in the Faculty of Nursing at the University of Windsor, Ontario, were aware of increasing levels of concern about patient safety[1-3] and calls to improve quality and safety education for nurses, including challenges to the profession from the Robert Wood Johnson Foundation (RWJF)–funded initiative, Quality and Safety Education for Nurses (QSEN).[4-6] Hospital clinical partners were engaged in efforts to reduce medication errors, but nursing faculty members had not been involved, even though they supervised learners in those settings. The University of Windsor faculty committee decided to work with their clinical partners to reduce the risk of patient harm from medication errors committed by students.[7]

With nurses and pharmacists from local hospitals, these faculty members initiated a collaborative Medication Safety Committee that has been meeting every 6–8 weeks for the last 3 years. By pulling together people concerned with patient care, system performance, and professional development, a number of outcomes were achieved.

- The medication administration policy for students was revised to incorporate current knowledge about high reliability systems and safe practice. Discussions about medication safety among committee members led to a reduction in the number of students per faculty member who administer medications during a clinical day.
- Error reports were discussed at each meeting, resulting in the development of standard operating procedures for students and clinical instructors that clearly outline the required steps in a safe medication administration process.
- At each meeting, information on new hospital policies, practices, and

equipment were shared, allowing faculty to prepare clinical instructors and incorporate new practices in simulated and laboratory learning scenarios.

- Hospitals actively encouraged error reporting so they could identify system vulnerabilities. The faculty adapted this strategy and designed an error reporting process to match the data captured by hospitals.
- A confusing aspect of the design of the computerized medication administration records (CMAR) emerged as a common error-prone condition for students. The committee proposed and accomplished a redesign of the hospital system CMAR.

In the faculty members' words:

> This hospital-academic partnership has been a win-win. Plans are underway to include students in medication reconciliation by teaching them to conduct a Best Possible Medication History interview, thus allowing our students to be active participants in improving safety in our hospitals and ensuring they are competent in this important safety practice when they graduate. Although the focus of our efforts continues to evolve, all members have eagerly taken on the challenges of this work, recognizing its importance in preparing tomorrow's nurses and contributing to the safety of the patients we serve.[8]

In an ideal world, this type of story would be common ... a source of energy and joy in health professionals' daily lives. Sadly, however, it is rare. In this chapter, we explore forces that diminish the extent to which nurses take into account each point of the triangle[9] (improving patient care, improving system performance, and improving professional development) as they work in separate spheres toward separate and unlinked aims. We also describe features of the QSEN initiative that served as catalysts for better linking the points of the triangle, and, in so doing, created opportunities, as in the story given here, for more sustainable sources of energy for improvement in each of the three domains.

Why "Windsor Experiences" Are Rare

The Professional Development Corner

Faculty

Taken together, faculties of nursing (across community colleges and universities) in the United States are the best-educated group of nurses in the country. By and large, they possess almost sole authority for the professional identity formation and development of students. When nursing education moved out of hospitals into academic institutions during the 1950s through to the 1970s, faculty members began earning graduate degrees commensurate with other faculties and were organized in departments within university administrative structures reporting to deans, provosts, and presidents. Unlike their medical school faculty counterparts who retained accountability for medical practice in academic health centers, nursing faculty members were (and are) generally isolated from accountability for nursing practice, population health, or health-care system performance. A few universities experimented with clinical and academic accountabilities for nurses (notably Rush University and the University of Rochester), but the experiments did not persist over time.[10] As faculty members sought (and were judged by) collegiate institutional rewards for teaching, research and service, fewer engaged in nursing practice.

When faculty members are isolated from clinical practice, what they teach may not be updated sufficiently to reflect current practice. Furthermore, because faculty members are not accountable for health care system performance, new models of teaching (such as dedicated education units[11]) are rarely evaluated in terms of their impact on patient or system outcomes.[3]

Calls to transform nursing education[12] to accomplish better integration of classroom and clinical education and ensure that new graduates acquire the clinical reasoning and ethical comportment required for nursing practice have attracted national attention. With practitioners and faculty members occupying narrowly defined roles at distinct corners of the triangle, partnerships among faculty and clinicians are critical to this transformation. Without the "Windsor experience" of drawing partners together to improve patient care and system performance, faculty members are no more than guests in health care settings, with limited opportunities for the types of engagement or leadership that might improve professional development as well as health and health care.

In summary, among the best-educated group of nurses, only a small percentage understand current issues related to each point of the triangle, and fewer still envision or embrace concurrent commitments to improving patient care, system performance, and professional development. Occasionally, vision and energy for spanning boundaries to improve all three corners come from nursing leaders who have moved between academic and practice settings as they built their careers. Adjunct clinical faculty members who are expert clinicians and preceptors of students sometimes provide strong role models for triangle commitments. In most settings, however, there are few, if any, positions or institutional rewards for nurses whose focus of attention spreads beyond the boundaries of one point of the triangle.

Scientists

One subgroup of faculty, the scientists who comprise the tenure-track faculties of research-intensive universities and academic health centers have only recently been incentivized by funders such as the National Institutes of Health (the revised Clinical and Translational Science Awards) and the Veteran's Administration Quality Scholars program (VAQS) to engage with communities of interest so that science will be "translated" into impact on improving health and health care. Nonetheless, the gaps remain wide between those accountable for comparative effectiveness and translational science and those accountable for embedding and sustaining cultures that use new knowledge to improve health and health care.

Scientists are rewarded for a laser-like focus on their programs of research and scholarship through promotion and tenure, funded grant proposals, and income from patents, spin-off businesses, and consultant roles. Young scientists, in fact, are often encouraged to *avoid* expending time and energy on boundary spanning efforts to improve patient care, system performance, or even professional development. It remains to be seen whether new incentives from funders will be sufficient to attract scientists to commitments beyond their focused area of scientific expertise.

Nurse scientists are similar to scientists in other fields with respect to the external incentives for staying focused on the generation of new knowledge while avoiding accountability for improving patient care, system performance or professional development. They differ in that nursing is a profession that is comparatively new to science. Some schools still have tenured faculty members who did not expect and were not prepared for scientific careers. The pressure on schools of nursing and individual scientists to excel in science in order to maintain credibility within the university and scientific world is great. Without alternate incentives, nurse scientists have strong motivations for maintaining a singular focus on the generation of knowledge, opting to work on improving one or more corners of the triangle only when their scientific findings improve the evidence base for a particular aspect of practice or education.

Individual/Population Health and System Performance Corners

Clinicians

In practice, the best-educated nurses are those who qualify for licensure as advanced practice registered nurses (APRNs) – namely, nurse anesthetists, nurse midwives, nurse practitioners, and clinical nurse specialists. As in the education of other health professionals, APRN education is focused primarily on the care of individual patients, with minimal attention to the development of the knowledge, skills, and attitudes required for improving health and health care.[6]

In addition, APRNs are rarely exposed to role models who, within practices or through boundary-spanning efforts, work to simultaneously improve patient care, system performance, and professional development.

Beyond these challenges, APRNs face hurdles associated with reimbursement and state licensure laws:[13]

- Licensure laws or insurers may require physician supervision of APRN practice, resulting in added costs and more complex system processes (with no evidence of impact on quality of care[14]) thus creating obstacles to APRN leadership in improving access and quality while reducing costs of care.
- Data about APRN contributions to patient care and system performance outcomes are often merged with and attributed to physicians, thus making it impossible for APRNs (and society) to fully understand their contributions to health and health-care improvement.
- In most employment arrangements to date, APRNs are employees of physician practices or hospitals. The freedom to engage in the professional development of advanced practice nursing students may be denied or limited by employer preferences for contributions to patient care or the teaching of medical students and residents.

In total, these barriers are formidable. Examples of APRN practices that hold together aims to improve patient care, system performance, and professional development exist,[15,16] but as yet, they are rare.

Administrators

The best-educated nurses in administrative roles are those who have assumed ranks of directors of nursing or chief nursing officers, operations, or executive officers within individual hospitals or health systems. Together with hospital administrators and physicians, they are responsible for creating a work environment and culture that can reliably produce safe and high-quality patient care. As health systems seek to engage with communities in improving patient and population health, nurse executives are frequently the leaders in nurturing the cross-boundary relationships required for effective work.

Yet there are major barriers to finding strong commitments to all three corners of the triangle among nurse administrators and executives. First, nurse administrators and executives may have less decision-making power and influence in their administrative roles than physicians and hospital administrators. Such realities may motivate nurses to focus on excelling in one corner of the triangle rather than embracing the complexity of improving in all three domains.

More important, because salaries for nurses in administrative roles are considerably higher than for faculty, leaders who have achieved director or executive roles in practice settings are rarely enticed into faculty roles (even when they would enjoy greater exposure to and accountability for professional development). Apart from serving as preceptors for students when they were in staff nurse roles, they are likely to have contributed little to the development and evaluation of curricula, pedagogical methods, or new programs of study (academic or professional) in nursing. This lack of experience may be a contributing factor when administrators implore faculties to place greater emphasis on technical skill development while also decrying, "these students can't think," not acknowledging (or perhaps realizing) the polarity implied in their critiques.

As administrators assume accountability for the professional development of their nursing employees, they often offer little more than a focus on policy and procedure review, skill or competency check-offs, or sessions required by regulatory or accrediting bodies. Respectful and engaged relationships between academic and practice partners could improve the entire continuum of professional formation and development while almost certainly improving system performance and the patient experience of care as well.

What If Leaders Were Role Models for Linking Triangle Commitments?

The discussion above focuses on challenges the best-educated, most influential nurses face in committing to link all three corners of the triangle in their day-to-day work. In each role, incentives to excel in one commitment (patient care, system performance, or professional development) are strong. It takes time and effort to listen to colleagues within and outside the profession so that one develops a deep understanding of the issues affecting each area of commitment. It takes even more time to put that understanding to use, with others, to improve patient care, system performance, and professional development. Lacking robust incentives and deriving rewards from focusing solely in one corner, it simply doesn't happen.

What would it take to have new degree programs developed by faculty and deans in partnership or in honest dialogue with colleagues in practice? What would it take to have innovations and improvements in systems of care spread to classrooms and laboratory teaching as a matter of common practice? To have nursing leaders in practice and faculty roles contribute to the improvement of system performance, thus enhancing the impact of their voices in national health policy decisions and debates? Perhaps most important, what would it take to have the vast majority of nurses and nursing students see their most powerful role models as examples of professional comportment and leadership for holding triangle commitments in their own lives?

In the recent Institute of Medicine[14] report on the future of nursing, one of eight recommendations is, "Prepare and enable nurses to lead change to advance health." We propose that effective health-care leadership requires a deep understanding of the synergies to be gained by innovations aimed at simultaneously improving patient care, system performance and professional development; furthermore, that the likelihood of excelling as a leader in any corner of the triangle is enhanced by visible and earnest commitments to all three corners.

Centrifugal Forces Inherent in Professional Identity Formation and Development

Beyond the boundary-spanning challenges that accrue to nurses with roles and accountabilities for single corners of the triangle, there are also challenges associated with historical approaches to professional development within nursing (and other health professions).

Lack of Preparation for Team-Based Care

As nursing moved from hospitals into academic institutions, pressures to articulate the unique contributions of nursing to patient care and to establish programs of research to generate nursing knowledge became paramount. For decades, students learned nursing theories and nursing diagnoses, used the nursing process and created nursing care plans. They focused on identifying roles for members of the nursing care team in care delivery settings.

Although faculty worked hard to prepare the next generation of nurses for practice with a clear sense of what it means to be a professional nurse, an unintended consequence of this approach was that nurses entered the workforce with a limited view of how to work collaboratively with other disciplines or how to access information outside the field of nursing. Many became nurses without ever having had a single meaningful conversation with a physician about patient care. Teaching students a unique language for nursing helped define the boundaries of the profession but added barriers to effective communication with other members of the health care team (as well as patients and families). In sum, nursing (and all the other health professions) educated their students in professional silos, doing little to prepare them for the complexities of daily work that included both delivering *and continuously improving* the care of patients and the systems within which they worked.

Sole Focus on Preparation for Individual Patient Care

For decades, the focus of almost all of health professions education (including nursing) has been the care of individual patients.[17] In nursing, during the supervised practice experiences that constitute clinical education, when a student has the opportunity to provide care to more than one patient, the emphasis is often on getting the work done and organizing and prioritizing the required care. Rarely do students engage in assessing patterns, variation or outcomes across a group of patients (or settings), examining if the care provided in a particular microsystem is consistent with current standards and evidence, or considering what, how and when improvements can be made (and how to make them). When this does occur, it is commonly isolated from the actual provision of care and comprised of extremely time-limited projects.[3] As a result, it is not surprising that many nurses do not see improving care and system performance as an integral part of their work.

Challenges of Continuing Professional Development

Once nurses enter the workforce, many professional development activities reproduce the same problems.[18] For instance, conferences are organized in professional silos so that nurses hear only from other nurses and talk only to other nurses throughout the event. Presentations commonly focus on providing nursing-specific content knowledge on a particular patient condition (or new policy or protocol), findings from a nursing research study, or an innovative approach to nursing practice or education. Rarely are these development activities situated in practice and focused on improvement (in more than an abstract way).

An underlying assumption of this approach is that content knowledge alone (knowing that) is sufficient to improve care. This assumption is reinforced by systems of mandatory continuing education in many states that rely only on the hours of exposure to professional development rather than on the extent to which that learning contributes to the improvement of patient care or system performance. Furthermore, continuing education requirements are frequently met based on convenience (time and location of the offering, available staff coverage, deadline for submitting documentation of continuing education), with little attention by individuals or organizations to the intentional, progressive development of expertise over time and in all three corners of the triangle.

Boundary-Spanning Leadership

Batalden and Foster[9] challenged us to consider what might be gained if improvement efforts took into account the need for synergistic change in each corner of the triangle. Recently, Ernst and Chrobot-Mason[19] described research on the challenges for leaders who seek to manage boundaries in order to forge common ground and discover new frontiers. Their descriptions of boundary-spanning leadership – *the ability to create direction, alignment, and commitment across boundaries in service of a higher vision or goal*[20] – are consistent with the notion that health professionals could derive greater energy for and effectiveness in improving health and health care if all sectors were aligned towards a higher vision or goal, such as, meeting needs of patients and communities for high-value (higher quality and reliability, lower cost) health care.

In their research, Ernst and Chrobot-Mason[19] found five types of boundaries (*see* Table 10.1). The challenges to triangle commitments by nurses described above include all but one of these types of boundaries, leading to multiple opportunities (and need for) boundary-spanning activities.

TABLE 10.1 Boundary Types and Boundary-Spanning Practices

Types of Boundaries	Helpful Boundary-Spanning Practices
Vertical: across levels, rank, seniority, authority, power **Horizontal**: across functions, units, peers, expertise **Stakeholder**: at the interchange of an organization and its external partners, such as alliances, networks, value chains, customers, shareholders, advocacy groups, governments, communities **Demographic**: between diverse groups, including the full range of human diversity from gender and race to education and ideology **Geographic**: across distance, locations, cultures, regions, markets	**Buffering**: monitoring and protecting the flow of information and resources across groups to define boundaries and create intergroup safety **Reflecting**: representing distinct perspectives and facilitating knowledge exchange across groups to understand boundaries and foster intergroup respect **Connecting**: linking people and bridging divided groups to suspend boundaries and build intergroup trust **Mobilizing**: crafting common purpose and shared identity across groups to reframe boundaries and develop intergroup community **Weaving**: drawing out and integrating group differences within a larger whole to interlace boundaries and advance intergroup interdependence **Transforming**: bringing multiple groups together in emergent, new directions to cross-cut boundaries and enable intergroup reinvention

From Ernst and Chrobot-Mason.[19]

Table 10.1 displays the six practices proposed by Ernst and Chrobot-Mason[19] for developing competence in boundary-spanning leadership. Physicians have often equated "medical care" and "health care," claiming all of health care as their domain. Nurses have usually focused on the "whole" patient. With all of health care and the whole patient "claimed" by physicians and nurses, the stage is set for all health professionals to spend endless amounts of energy on the first practice – defining boundaries, effectively limiting attention to the several other constructive practices. The professional identities that result contribute to self-esteem and provide a sense of connection, belonging, and safety. Unfortunately, the boundaries also contribute to "us versus them" views of the world and many difficulties forging common ground to make the connections necessary for boundary-spanning leadership in service of higher aims.

It is beyond the scope of this chapter to fully describe the remaining five practices, but suffice it to say, if we are to succeed in reframing boundaries that include all corners of the triangle within and across health professions, nursing professional development needs to include distinctly new types of opportunities. Nurses, physicians, and others need to learn how to better understand, suspend, reframe, interlace, and transform boundaries to enable reinvention.[19]

Transforming Boundaries and Enabling Reinvention
• •

Opportunities for Boundary-Spanning

Over the last decade, there have been many examples of efforts to transform boundaries within the health-care field. Ideas from the Quality Chasm series of studies reported by the Institute of Medicine beginning with Kohn *et al.*[1] and the National Priorities Partnership project,[21] resulted in national efforts to improve health care (better patient experience of care, better system performance, and lower costs). Incentives for horizontal and stakeholder boundary spanning were even embedded in the US 2010 Patient Protection and Affordable Care Act.[22]

With respect to spanning professional boundaries, multiple calls were recently issued for greater attention to interprofessional team and team-based care,[23] interprofessional education,[14,24] and better use of the health-care workforce by using professionals to the full scope of their education and scope of practice.[14,25] Similarly, leaders within nursing called for a variety of mechanisms to incentivize boundary-spanning between education and practice.[10,26] During this time, the RWJF invested in a national initiative to improve quality and safety education for nurses (QSEN).

Quality and Safety Education for Nurses: Deriving Energy from Triangle Synergies

QSEN goals and strategies and examples of the initiative's initial impact on nursing education, licensure, and accreditation of nursing programs have been described elsewhere.[27] Although it is tempting to re-vision the rationale for QSEN strategies as if there were preconceived, conscious efforts to simultaneously improve patient care, system performance, and professional development, such was *not* the case. Nonetheless, a number of features of the initiative and its program elements served to highlight and provide incentives for the kind of triangle synergies exemplified in this chapter's opening story.

Envisioning the Work

The overarching QSEN goal (to alter the professional identity formation of nurses so that future nurses would possess the knowledge, skills, and attitudes needed to make continuous improvement of health and health care a part of their daily work) was, from the beginning, a goal that served to integrate commitments to improving patient care, system performance, and professional development. The work emerged from a learning community – the Dartmouth Summer Symposium (DSS) – comprised of nurse, physician, and hospital administrator leaders who describe themselves as *an interprofessional community of educators devoted to building knowledge for leading improvement in health care*. In annual week-long meetings (from 1995 to the present), the community struggled with how to attract faculty to engage in health-care improvement and develop the needed competencies in students. These efforts served to deepen each person's understanding of the corners of the triangle, including unique viewpoints that arose across professions.

A similar struggle affected leaders of the nursing and quality portfolios within the RWJF who were managing grants (e.g., *Transforming Care at the Bedside*[28]) where robust attempts to attract educators to the work of improving patient care quality and system performance had fallen well short of expectations. Their personal experience with the chasm between nurses concerned with professional development and those concerned with patient/population health and system performance provided the rationale needed for RWJF executives to provide almost 8 years of funding for six QSEN grants.

QSEN Leaders

Six of the twelve QSEN faculty leaders, including the principal investigator, were members of the DSS community.[26] Five of the twelve, including the principal investigator, had integrated various corners of the triangle within their personal careers – having served as leaders within both academic and health-care systems. As a result, the personal careers and commitments of QSEN leaders influenced the strategies designed to create synergy between improvements in professional development, patient/population health, and system performance.

Collectively, QSEN leaders knew the issues of each triangle corner in considerable depth and their networks included professional organizational leaders who represented the interests of nurses in each triangle corner – faculty members, clinicians, and administrators. As QSEN leaders worked to build will for a paradigm shift in quality and safety education, they used multiple opportunities – in speeches, workshops, and publications – to challenge the idea that one could be a leading health-care educator if one was not concerned about outcomes of care or system performance.

The Boundary-Spanning Composition of the QSEN Advisory Board

In addition to the faculty, QSEN leaders engaged an advisory board of leaders from organizations with responsibility for nursing licensure, certification, and accreditation of education programs. The design and implementation of the first two phases of QSEN funding were led by the faculty and advisory board acting together as one group. Two physician leaders from the DSS community and a leading nurse executive added perspectives that helped foster intergroup and cross-triangle respect and understanding, while providing fertile conversations about how to reframe boundaries in service of a higher mission.

The QSEN Learning Collaborative

One of the most effective strategies, in terms of developing nurses' capacity for boundary-spanning leadership, was the design of the QSEN Learning Collaborative.[29] To prepare for a widespread faculty development initiative, QSEN first needed to attract faculty innovators to develop, test, and disseminate teaching strategies for QSEN competency development. A nationwide call for proposals was issued to every school of nursing in the country. The call itself fostered awareness of the need for improvements in nursing education that could foster improvements in patient care and system performance. It also required that educators enter into conversations with their practice partners if they planned to seek one of 15 grant proposals that would be offered to schools selected to be QSEN Learning Collaborative participants.

Each school identified a team of four people who would participate in the national collaborative meetings and lead quality and safety education innovations in their settings. The teams were required to have a clinical setting partner in addition to a clinical teacher, a simulation/skills laboratory teacher, and a classroom teacher. As 15 teams from all types of nursing programs worked together as a Collaborative, they learned about each corner of the triangle, enriching their own triangle commitments through enhanced visions about what each person could do to improve patient care, system performance, and professional development. The collaboration of academic and clinical partners across organizations during the generative brainstorming phases of the work of the Collaborative enriched the teaching strategies that emerged as well as the relationships between academic and practice partners.

In the qualitative portions of the evaluation of the Collaborative, participants commented frequently on the value of the improved academic-practice partnerships that resulted from QSEN work.[24,29] Indeed, Collaborative teams gained new energy for improving patient outcomes, system performance, and professional development from working together, resulting in reports of professional joy in response to making an impact in service of important goals. While it is too early to determine the long-term effect of QSEN on the pervasive forces described earlier (i.e., the academic-practice gap), it has clearly drawn attention to the joy and energy participants derive from transforming their work to keep the corners of the triangle together in service of higher goals.

Interprofessional Incentives

From the start, one of the 10 QSEN leaders was chosen specifically because of her expertise in fostering interprofessional learning related to quality improvement. Another leader worked on the QSEN competency "teamwork and collaboration." They were role models in developing teaching strategies and also challenged Collaborative members to change curricula in ways that would prepare future health professionals for effective teamwork and team-based care.[24] Furthermore, both physicians on the QSEN advisory board participated in Collaborative meetings in ways that reframed and interlaced professional boundaries in the service of improving patient/population health, system performance, and professional development. In addition, in the many opportunities they had to speak to national gatherings of nursing faculties, QSEN leaders openly questioned the notion that nurses could be part of high-performing patient-centered health-care teams if every member of the team spoke a different language in naming problems, treatments, and outcomes (something taught to most nursing students over the past few decades). Each of these actions stimulated innovations to support interprofessional education and improved teamwork and collaboration in practice.

QSEN was about to enter its third phase of work (a national faculty development initiative) when an opportunity arose to partner with the VAQS program.[30] After 10 years of funding for a physician quality improvement scholars program, VAQS leaders were exploring the option of expanding the program to nurses. Because the VA did not employ nursing faculties in the same way as physician faculties, there were barriers to paying nursing faculty mentors for work in an interprofessional program. With the support of funding from RWJF, QSEN was able to partner with the VAQS program to provide funding for nursing faculty members. For the first time, nursing pre- and postdoctoral scholars had incentives for interprofessional learning and engagement in quality improvement science. The results have been so successful, from the VA's perspective, that the barriers to full inclusion of nursing faculty have been removed, and, beginning in 2012, nursing faculty salaries will transfer from QSEN to VAQS funding.

Conclusion

By creating synergies among improving care, system performance, and professional development, professionals, organizations, and national initiatives like VAQS and QSEN help enable reinvention of strategies for achieving higher goals than those based in narrow, inherited, and individual-focused views of nursing (and other health professions). To respond to the quality and safety challenges in contemporary health care, a strong body of disciplinary knowledge, while necessary, is not sufficient. Bold changes in the ways nurses are prepared for practice and continue to learn across their careers must include meaningful practice-based, interprofessional experiences that focus on both the theoretical and phronetic knowledge needed to persistently improve health and health-care systems.

The triangle provides a way to rethink the working relationships among nursing teachers, scientists, practitioners, and administrators. For instance, keeping the corners of the triangle together, faculty members would be role models for commitments to professional development, individual patient care *and* system performance wherever clinical supervision was provided. Scientists would be concerned about generating knowledge *and* improving system capabilities to reliably move new knowledge into practice. Dissertations could include sections on how the study contributed to improved care, system performance, and professional development. Promotion and tenure cases could be restructured so that a junior faculty member's scholarship was assessed by the impact it had on each of the corners. Importantly, these changes would not just represent a new technical element to be addressed by candidates. Rather, they would reflect the discipline's sharp focus on altering the professional identity of nurses, whether in academic or practice settings, such that improving care, system performance, and professional development were as integral to nursing identity as honesty, integrity, knowledge, and care.

The expression of such new identities will take many forms. Some nurses will develop triangle expertise by spending time in roles that focus on each corner, but their experiences over time will generate the insights needed to improve the whole. Others will develop their commitments by serving in professional or inter-professional organizations that increase their exposure to and impact on issues across triangle boundaries. Many will create partnerships across organizational boundaries in order to better meet societal needs for improved patient/population health, system performance, and professional development.

The path for each nurse will be easier if professional development (initial training and continuing education) provides a platform for triangle commitments as part of the normal preparation for and advancement in professional life, if professional regulatory mechanisms (licensure, certification, and accreditation of nursing programs) integrate the corners through their requirements and rewards, if boundary-spanning leadership is a prerequisite for nursing and health care leader roles, and if health professionals earn rewards and incentives for triangle expertise commensurate with those obtained for expertise in a single corner. In such a future, the story of the University of Windsor and its partners will be one of many, and health professionals will find new sources of energy for improving health and health care.

References

1. Kohn LT, Corrigan JM, Donaldson MS, editors. *To Err is Human: building a safer health system.* Washington, DC: National Academies Press; 2000.
2. Aspden P, Wolcott J, Bootman L, *et al.*, editors. *Preventing Medication Errors.* Washington, DC: National Academies Press; 2006.
3. Cook M, Ironside PM, Ogrinc G. Mainstreaming quality and safety: a reformulation of quality

and safety education for health professions students. *Qual Saf Health Care*. 2011; **20**(Suppl. 1): 179–82.

4. Cronenwett L, Sherwood G, Barnsteiner J, *et al*. Quality and safety education for nurses. *Nurs Outlook*. 2007; **55**(3): 122–31.

5. Cronenwett L, Sherwood G, Gelmon SB. Improving quality and safety education: the QSEN Learning Collaborative. *Nurs Outlook*. 2009; **57**(6): 304–12.

6. Cronenwett L, Sherwood G, Pohl J, *et al*. Quality and safety education for advanced nursing practice. *Nurs Outlook*. 2009; **57**(6): 338–48.

7. Freeman M, Dennison S. *Safe Medication Administration: from policy to practice*. Proceedings of the 2011 QSEN National Forum, 2011, June 1; Milwaukee, WI. Available at: www.qsen. org/docs/2011_conference/QSEN_2011_Freeman.pdf (accessed November 22, 2011).

8. Freeman M, Dennison S. Partnering to support safe medication practices with nursing students. 2011. Unpublished manuscript.

9. Batalden P. The evolutionary beginnings of the model. In: Batalden P, Foster T, editors. *Sustainably Improving Health Care: creatively linking care outcomes, system performance, and professional development*. London: Radcliffe Publishing; 2012.

10. Malloch K, Porter-O'Grady T. Innovations in academic and practice partnerships: new collaborations within existing models. *Nurs Admin Quart*. 2011; **35**(4): 300–05.

11. Warner JR, Moscato SR. Innovative approach to clinical education: dedicated education units. In: Ard N, Valiga TM, editors. *Clinical Nursing Education: current reflections*. New York, NY: National League for Nursing; 2009. pp. 59–70.

12. Benner P, Sutphen M, Leonard V, *et al*. *Educating Nurses: a call for radical transformation*. San Francisco, CA: Jossey-Bass; 2010.

13. Pohl JM, Hanson C, Newland JA, *et al*. Unleashing nurse practitioners' potential to deliver primary care and lead teams. *Health Affairs*. 2010; **29**(5): 900–05.

14. Institute of Medicine. *The Future of Nursing: leading change, advancing health*. Washington, DC: National Academies Press; 2011.

15. Flinter M. Residency programs for primary care nurse practitioners in federally qualified health centers: a service perspective. *Online J Issues Nurs*. 2005; **10**(3). Available at: www.nursingworld.org/MainMenuCategories/ANAMarketplace/ANAPeriodicals/OJIN/TableofContents/Volume102005/No3Sept05/tpc28_516029.html (accessed November 22, 2011).

16. Barkauskas VH, Pohl JM, Tanner C, *et al*. Quality of care in nurse-managed health centers. *Nurs Admin Quart*. 2011; **35**(1): 34–43.

17. IOM (Institute of Medicine). *Health professions education: a bridge to quality*. Washington, DC: National Academies Press; 2003.

18. Ironside PM. Safeguarding patients through continuing competency. *J Cont Educ Nurs*. 2008; **39**(2): 92–4.

19. Ernst C, Chrobot-Mason D. *Boundary Spanning Leadership: six practices for solving problems, driving innovation, and transforming organizations*. New York, NY: McGraw Hill; 2011.

20. Yip J, Ernst C, Campbell M. *Boundary Spanning Leadership: mission critical perspectives from the executive suite*. Center for Creative Leadership organizational leadership white paper. Greensboro, NC: Center for Creative Leadership; 2009.

21. National Priorities Partnership. *National Priorities and Goals: aligning our efforts to transform America's Healthcare*. Washington, DC: National Quality Forum; 2008. Available at: http:// nationalprioritiespartnership.org/uploadedFiles/NPP/08-253-NQF%20ReportLo%5B6%5D. pdf (accessed November 22, 2011).

22. Office of Legislative Counsel of the US House of Representatives. *Compilation of Patient Protection and Affordable Care Act*. Available at: http://docs.house.gov/energycommerce/ppacacon.pdf (accessed November 22, 2011).

23. Interprofessional Education Collaborative. *Core Competencies for Interprofessional Collaborative Practice: report of an expert panel*. Washington, DC: Interprofessional Education

Collaborative; 2011. Available at: www.aacn.nche.edu/Education/pdf/IPECReport.pdf (accessed November 22, 2011).

24. Barnsteiner J, Disch J, Hall L, *et al.* Promoting interprofessional education. *Nurs Outlook.* 2007; **55**(3): 144–50.

25. Cunningham R. *Tapping the Potential of the Health Care Workforce: scope-of-practice and payment policies for advanced practice nurses and physician assistants.* National Health Policy Forum Background Paper No. 76. July 6, 2010. Available at: www.nhpf.org/library/details. cfm/2808 (accessed November 22, 2011).

26. Cronenwett LR. The future of nursing education: summary and conclusions. In: Institute of Medicine. *The Future of Nursing: leading change, advancing health.* Washington, DC: National Academies Press; 2011. pp. 467–82.

27. Cronenwett L. A national initiative: quality and safety education for nurses (QSEN). In: Sherwood G, Barnsteiner J, editors. *Quality and Safety in Nursing: a competency approach to improving outcomes.* Hoboken, NJ: Wiley-Blackwell; 2012. pp. 49–64.

28. Hassmiller SB, Bolton LB. The development of TCAB: an initiative to improve patient care and nursing retention. *Am J Nurs.* 2009; **109**(11 Suppl.): 4.

29. Cronenwett L, Sherwood G, Gelmon SB. Improving quality and safety education: the QSEN learning collaborative. *Nurs Outlook.* 2009; **57**(6): 304–12.

30. Splaine ME, Ogrinc G, Gilman SC, *et al.* The Department of Veterans Affairs National Quality Scholars Fellowship Program: experience from 10 years of training quality scholars. *Acad Med.* 2009; **84**(12): 1741–8.

Collaborative Improvement of Cancer Services in Southeastern Sweden

Striving for Better Patient and Population Health, Better Care, and Better Professional Development

Johan Thor, Charlotte Lundgren, Paul Batalden,
Boel Andersson Gäre, Göran Henriks, Rune Sjödahl,
and Felicia Gabrielsson Järhult

Who is interested in improving health care services related to colon cancer – from preventive services, through early detection, diagnostic, therapeutic, and rehabilitation services to end-of-life care? In the case of southeastern Sweden, the answer just might be *everyone*! In this chapter, we aim to bring the triangle model to life in the context of a demonstration project to improve colon cancer services for one million residents in southeastern Sweden that involves "healthcare professionals, patients and their families, researchers, payers, [leaders,] planners and educators,"[1] spanning multiple organizational boundaries.

How, then, might the triangle model apply in this setting, with universal access to health care services for the entire population in a geographic area? We will first describe some distinctive aspects of the Swedish health care system, and then describe a specific initiative to improve colon cancer services for all one million residents in three counties in southeastern Sweden, including a case study of one aspect of that initiative. The chapter concludes with reflections on the applicability of the triangle model, as well as how its embodiment may be influenced by health system characteristics.

Health Care the Swedish Way

Health-care services in Sweden are "aimed at assuring the entire population of good health and of care on equal terms." Care is to be provided "with respect for the equal dignity of all human beings and for the dignity of the individual. Priority for health and medical care shall be given to the person whose need of care is greatest."[2-4] Health care is democratically governed at three levels: (1) *national* (mostly regulation, oversight, and technology assessment); (2) *regional* (most health care); and (3) *local* (mostly social care, including services for the elderly and some home health care) levels. The tax-based financing and provision of comprehensive "cradle to grave" health-care services is the responsibility of the 20 county councils and regions and of the 290 municipalities that comprise Swedish society. Historically, county councils owned and operated most health-care facilities. Today, greater diversity of provider arrangements is emerging, particularly in primary care where cooperatives and for-profit entrepreneurs operate a growing proportion of primary care centers on a contract basis with the county councils. Irrespective of provider structures, the same fundamental objectives of the health-care system apply.

For purposes of accountability and improvement, Open Comparison reports on Swedish health-care performance have been published annually since 2006.[5] They emphasize patient outcomes – the upper left corner in the triangle model – and gather data from national quality registers and other national data sources. The units of analysis are predominantly county councils, but include individual hospitals and municipalities. Indicators cover a wide range of conditions including:

- *policy-related avoidable mortality* – diagnoses and causes of death (lung cancer, esophageal cancer, cirrhosis of the liver and motor vehicle accidents) that can be affected by broad policy interventions, such as campaigns for smoking cessation and improved alcohol habits
- *health-care-related avoidable mortality* – avoidable deaths from diagnoses that can be affected by medical interventions (e.g., diabetes, appendicitis, stroke, gallstone disease, and cervical cancer)
- *avoidable hospitalization* – hospitalization that can be avoided if patients receive proper outpatient care; specifically for patients with diabetes; heart failure; chronic obstructive lung disease; bleeding ulcers; diarrhea; inflammatory diseases of female pelvic organs; pyelitis; and ear, nose, and throat infection
- *structure-adjusted health care costs per capita*
- *cost per diagnosis-related group point for hospitals*
- colon cancer relative 5-year survival rates (*see* Figure 11.1; note that the three counties in this effort, Kalmar, Jönköping, and Östergötland, are all below the national average).[6]

Collaborative Improvement of Cancer Services in Southeastern Sweden

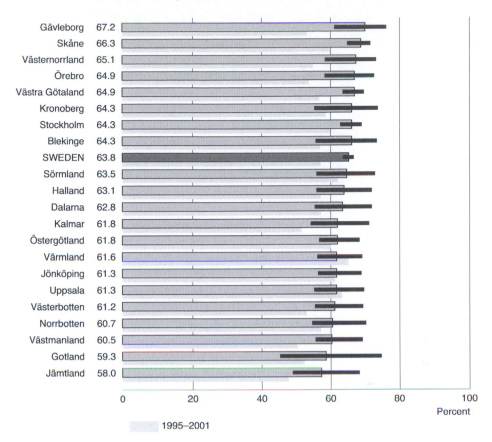

County/Region	Value
Gävleborg	67.2
Skåne	66.3
Västernorrland	65.1
Örebro	64.9
Västra Götaland	64.9
Kronoberg	64.3
Stockholm	64.3
Blekinge	64.3
SWEDEN	63.8
Sörmland	63.5
Halland	63.1
Dalarna	62.8
Kalmar	61.8
Östergötland	61.8
Värmland	61.6
Jönköping	61.3
Uppsala	61.3
Västerbotten	61.2
Norrbotten	60.7
Västmanland	60.5
Gotland	59.3
Jämtland	58.0

1995–2001

FIGURE 11.1 Relative 5-year survival rates for women diagnosed with colon cancer, 2002–08, by county/region[6]

The broad social commitment to universal access and equality in health helps explain the concerns that arise when health care does not serve everyone equally well, as is the case in cancer services. The Commission of Inquiry on a National Cancer Strategy highlighted, in its final report,[7] Sweden's ranking in the middle among its European Union peers with regard to the general public's satisfaction with health and medical care in general, and widespread concerns regarding "inadequate continuity and fragmentary care with long waiting lists, resulting in anxiety and uncertainty."[7] It also quoted projections of increases in cancer incidence and prevalence – by 130% for men and 70% for women, with about half of it due to demographic changes – over the next 20 years. It articulated concerns over escalating costs of cancer care and over challenges in developing the health-care workforce's capacity and competence – concerns corresponding with the bottom and upper right corners of the triangle model (concerning better care and better professional development). The Commission advocated the pursuit of several opportunities for improvement, including:

- increase investments in prevention – the most significant element in reducing cancer morbidity and mortality
- improve the generation and dissemination of knowledge in cancer care and prevention
- develop comprehensive cancer services
- make cancer services more patient-focused to better meet patients' information needs, to strengthen their sense that their wishes and expectations are met, and to enhance patients' confidence in the services offered
- reduce differences between population groups in terms of the risk of developing and dying from cancer by adapting services to the increasingly heterogeneous population and turning the tide of increasing social inequalities.

The Commission proposed a program of 3-year demonstration projects to generate ideas for accomplishing these improvements. We report here on the largest of the four funded projects, which involves an entire region: three adjacent county councils – Jönköping, Kalmar, and Östergötland – form the southeastern health care region in Sweden (*see* Figure 11.2), covering just over 1 million (out of Sweden's 9.5 million) residents,[8] with an area roughly equal to Vermont and New Hampshire combined.[9] While each county council is responsible for its residents' health care, the three counties cooperate on regional health-care issues including

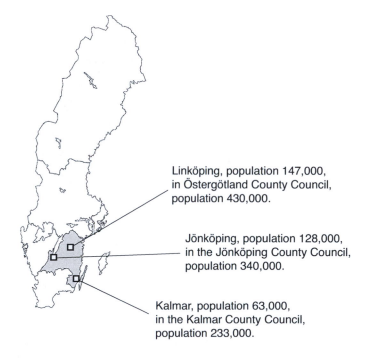

Linköping, population 147,000, in Östergötland County Council, population 430,000.

Jönköping, population 128,000, in the Jönköping County Council, population 340,000.

Kalmar, population 63,000, in the Kalmar County Council, population 233,000.

FIGURE 11.2 The southeastern health care region in Sweden (source: Statistics Sweden, population data, September 30, 2011)

tertiary care offered at the University Hospital in Linköping, Östergötland, home to the Faculty of Health Sciences, which includes the only medical school in the region. Medical students go on clinical rotations throughout the region, along with students in nursing and allied health professions, who are also trained at the universities in Jönköping and Kalmar. The three counties collaboratively fund clinical and health services research in the region through the Medical Research Council of Southeast Sweden.

Pilot Project on Improving Services for Colon Cancer

Leaders and faculty from around the region met and designated subject matter experts and improvement facilitators to support the improvement efforts. Drawing on extensive local improvement experience[10–12] and on the Breakthrough Collaborative model,[13–17] the work was designed with recurring regional "learning seminars" – convening multiprofessional clinical teams and public health staff – and intervening periods for action "at home." At the first seminar, a patient from the region, who had recently been treated for colon cancer, shared his story with the assembled professionals – a recurring approach in this demonstration project, and an example of how patients and family members can truly be included in the "everyone" of the triangle model.

After the broad objectives and agreements were settled, participating teams were encouraged to examine current practice patterns and begin to pursue opportunities for improvement. They were advised in particular to draw on knowledge-based methods for improvement, to use measurement and process orientation, to involve patients and their loved ones, and to collaborate in communities of practice.[18]

Recognizing that health care is a geographically distributed service, the program team charged with managing the project was complemented by one team in each county, bringing together clinical teams from some of the two to three hospitals in each county and the approximately 130 primary health care centers in the region. In addition, a public health team formed, with staff from each of the counties to assess and develop preventive and other public health measures in the region. Similarly, a team focused on measurement related to colon cancer services and their improvement was formed. Another team was formed to address the use of information technology and its improvement in colon (and other) cancer services. A professor emeritus of surgery in Linköping led collaborative clinical practice studies regarding colon cancer care and visited all departments of surgery in the region. Finally, a group of regional health services researchers (including some authors of this chapter) formed a team to document and study the demonstration project as it unfolded (*see* Figure 11.3). This multidisciplinary

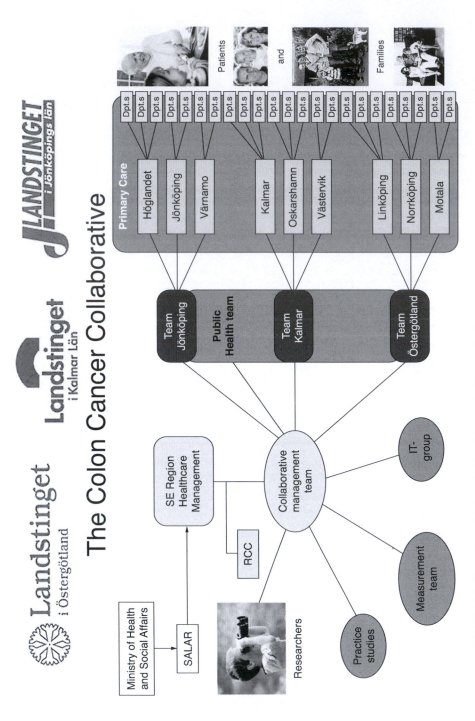

FIGURE 11.3 Overview of actors in the demonstration project

and broad-based approach reflects the commitment to understanding outcomes, working closely with the multiple systems that patients and families encounter, including the public health system, and built-in opportunities for professional development in the form of ongoing, collaborative learning seminars.

Context

Actions by the Regional Political, Managerial, and Clinical Leadership

In parallel with the colon cancer demonstration project, the regional health-care leadership established its Regional Cancer Center (RCC) based in Linköping. Part of a national expansion of support for cancer services and surveillance, the RCCs in each region are intended to:

- reduce the risk for developing cancer
- improve the quality of care, from a distinct patient perspective
- prolong survival and enhance the quality of life following a cancer diagnosis
- reduce regional disparities in survival
- reduce disparities in cancer incidence and survival among different popula tion groups.[19]

Governed by a board with politicians from each of the county councils, the RCC is directed by regional health care executives and its own management team. Early on, the political board issued a vision statement for regional cancer services: *"I get the care and support that I need, when I need it."* It also made the following promises to all residents and patients in the region:

- All cancer patients can start treatment within 4 weeks.
- All cancer patients are offered best practice diagnostic and therapeutic services.
- All cancer patients are well informed and actively involved throughout the care process.
- All cancer patients at the end of life receive equally good palliative care regard-less of their location.
- All cancer patients are offered the best possible health-promoting services and well-functioning screening programs.
- The Southeast Regional Cancer Center prioritizes patient-related research in the cancer field.

While obviously not limited to colon cancer, these promises provided powerful direction for the demonstration project. The promises are visionary, in light of the fact that they are not yet a reality for many cancer patients in Sweden, in the southeast region or elsewhere.

A Multicomponent Action Plan

The program team developed and disseminated a plan of action – publicly available on the Internet, with continuous updates – which reveals the approach taken: to seek improvement through multiple parallel efforts. In the action plan, there is a goal and a person in charge of the work stated for each of its 43 areas. One area, for example, is reducing the proportion of patients who have metastasized cancer at the time of diagnosis. The first phase of the work has included review of medical records for patients in the region with such advanced disease, led by two senior clinicians. Another area concerns application of practices to optimize perioperative care – for example, the Enhanced Recovery After Surgery model.[20] A third example is efforts to promote smoking cessation in order to prevent smoking-related complications such as impaired wound healing.[21] Let us now take a closer look at some of the actions in the demonstration project, as a foundation for considering the applicability of the triangle model.

Clinical Practice Assessment

In order to better understand regional colon cancer services' performance, a pilot project reviewed medical records – using a global trigger tool[22] and a "patient perspective protocol" regarding the care process – for five randomly selected patients who had undergone treatment for colon cancer in 2010 at each of the regions' seven hospitals offering such services. Out of the 35 patients (16 men, 19 women, with median age 71 years), nine patients (26%) were emergency admissions.[23] The record review revealed that nearly half (46%) of the patients suffered some kind of adverse event that prolonged their hospital stay or required various measures; only 35% of cases received therapy within 30 days of their first health care contact; the median time span was 46 days. The findings clearly indicated room for improvement in the areas of outcomes and system performance.

With inspiration from a collaborative improvement effort targeting colon surgery more broadly,[24] clinical leaders in surgery, oncology, and palliative care have articulated a regional best practice guide for colon cancer. It includes giving structured information to patients and their loved ones, referral to a multidisciplinary team treatment conference, thrombosis prophylaxis for more than 10 days, and regular assessment of symptoms – including pain – using validated instruments. Adherence to these practices and their impact will be assessed using the same approach that was used in the pilot study.

Early Detection

While the American College of Gastroenterology argues that colonoscopy "is the preferred method of screening for colorectal cancer [and] considers colonoscopy the 'gold standard' for colorectal screening,"[25] Sweden has not (yet) adopted general screening for colorectal cancer by way of regular colonoscopies because of skepticism about the evidence base, safety, and cost-effectiveness of such screening programs.[26] Concerns over the health-care system's capacity to perform sufficient numbers of colonoscopies have also influenced the policy. Plans have been considered for over a decade (but not adopted) to introduce population-based screening with fecal occult blood testing, with tests disseminated and returned through regular mail, in peak incidence age groups. A clinical trial of such an approach is currently underway elsewhere in Sweden. National policy may change depending on the findings from this trial, and scientific advances elsewhere.

So, without population-based screening, what might clinicians in the southeastern region do to detect colorectal cancers as early as possible? A group of four nurses and four family physicians (FPs), with support from the primary care research and development unit in Jönköping, took on this question from their vantage point, seeking to develop ways to optimize the chance of early detection. One challenge in primary care is to distinguish signs and symptoms of cancer from the "noise" of much more common and benign causes. In a population-based survey,[27] respondents reported the following incidence of symptoms potentially indicative of colon cancer over the preceding 3 months: feeling tired (35.8%); stomach pain (23.6%); diarrhea (10.0%); constipation (5.8%); poor appetite (5.3%). With an incidence of three cases per 10 000 residents, a Swedish FP will, on average, come across one patient with colorectal cancer once every 3 years. The group developed the "Stålhammar Score"[28] to manage this challenge. In short, patients aged 50 years or over who seek care with certain symptoms – for example, "sub-ileus (intermittent, increasing abdominal pain)" – are considered high risk and are seen within 3 days by their FP who initiates the assessment and refers the patient to the department of surgery where the remaining diagnostic workup is expediently coordinated.

To validate their Stålhammar Score, the group performed a pilot test in four primary health care centers, responsible for 31 700 residents, during a 4-week period. They also reviewed the medical records of 50 patients who had undergone surgery for colorectal cancer in 2010, and applied the score to their pre-diagnostic history. During the pilot test period, the nurses and doctors involved identified eight high-risk patients according to the score. Extrapolating to all primary care in the Jönköping County Council, the group predicted that some 1000 patients would be identified with a high-risk score each year, 60–70 of whom would turn out to have colorectal cancer. In other words, about 1 in 15 such high-risk score patients would actually have colorectal cancer. Of the 50 patients operated on during the preceding year, 42 (84%) would have been identified by the Stålhammar Score. The group concluded, based on this small-scale test, that the Stålhammar Score might contribute to early detection and a better prognosis, although these findings need to be confirmed in larger studies. They also reason that population-based screening, if introduced, may be more effective at reducing mortality from colorectal cancer.

Toward Better Diagnostic Services

As with all breakthrough collaboratives, a key ingredient in the demonstration project is learning from the approach and experience of participating peers. The Kalmar County Council shared an approach for expedient diagnostic assessment of patients with suspected gastrointestinal cancer, developed prior to the demonstration project. Rather than taking a traditional, sequential approach with multiple separate diagnostic steps, patients referred for speedy assessment undergo all necessary tests as in-patients during 2–3 days at the hospital in Oskarshamn. In a similar vein, a group of clinicians and managers in the Östergötland County Council set out to enhance the diagnostic services there, by developing the *Abdominal Cancer Diagnostic Unit*.

On October 3, 2011, a cross-departmental pilot project went live at the Linköping University Hospital. There, a multidisciplinary and multiprofessional team began its work to test how an innovative clinical microsystem could improve the care of patients suffering from gastrointestinal malignancies. Three mornings a week, four doctors (two gastrointestinal oncological surgeons, one oncologist, and one palliative care specialist) sit down with two nurses (one specialized in surgery and one specialized in palliative care) for half an hour in order to discuss referrals and decide on how to proceed with further assessment.

The pilot project, named ACDU (the Abdominal Cancer Diagnostic Unit), was set up to engage two primary health care centers (PHCCs). The family practitioners at the two centers care for a population of 27 000 inhabitants. The idea behind the project is to create opportunities for dialogue between the participating PHCCs and the specialized hospital practitioners regarding the management of patients suffering from various symptoms from the gastrointestinal tract, some of who are developing abdominal cancer.

At least four features distinguish this project from many others aiming at quality improvement:
1. no set protocol
2. grass-roots initiative
3. innovative set up of microsystem
4. presence of non-medical personnel.

The most striking feature is that there was no set protocol regulating the ACDU's work when the project went live. Instead, there was a frame (the participating disciplines, the participating professionals, the time dedicated for meetings, the agreement with the two participating PHCCs and goals stated by the County Council's democratic board) to guide the stakeholders. The rest was for the participating professionals in the project to decide upon: inclusion and exclusion criteria, meeting routines, division of labor and so forth.

Another salient feature was the way the project came about: it started as a true grass-roots initiative. During the initial formation of the demonstration project, three persons discovered that they had independently come to the same conclusion: insufficient communication with and about the patients and a lack of flexibility to meet individual patients' needs caused unnecessary harm both to the patients and the professionals. Informal discussions revealed their consensus on the problem description and a willingness to explore change, culminating in this new model for collaboration.

The third significant feature of the project is the innovative setup of the microsystem. Traditionally, the clinicians from surgery, oncology, and palliative care rarely meet face to face. The qualities of face-to-face communication – enhanced trust, shared decision making, and greater accountability to one another and the organizations involved – rarely evolve in the rhythm of everyday clinical work, but they have had the chance to do so in the ACDU.

Another ingredient in the innovative setup is the presence of three nonclinical team members whose roles are to facilitate the work of the clinical staff. An administrator brought knowledge and skill of navigating and adapting information technology systems, which freed up clinical staff time. A clinical guideline coordinator worked to integrate the needs of the ACDU with the rest of the health care system and a social scientist and communications researcher (CL, author of this case report) helped guide a process of continuous reflection.

Three months into the project, ACDU staff members report a steep learning curve and a number of evolutionary crises. A major finding has been the exposure of problems in the surrounding health care system, discussed later in this section. It is also clear that when clinicians are under pressure it can be easy to revert to prior suboptimal behaviors and routines. When faced with this, participants have found it helpful to challenge each other's thinking by highlighting the need to "be better than we used to be or how we used to think." Challenging assumptions in daily work has changed the direction of the team's discussion and often has led to innovative approaches to care. The team members repeatedly make the point that this is one of the most important outcomes of the interdisciplinary discussions: they continually challenge each other's assumptions about the best solution for each patient. The ACDU can be described as a site of learning as well as a site of fruitful and high-quality clinical work, which explicitly considers the role of different systems in the care of individual patients. The team members report that their discussions have provided many insights, which have in turn affected their interactions, leading to an increased and more holistic understanding of how the participating disciplines and professions interpret various symptoms and how they think about how to respond. The team members also report moving from acting as a representative of one's discipline and/or profession on the team to acting more as a full team member of a team with shared, mutual accountability for actions in and outside of the team meetings. This can easily be traced in recordings of team meetings; early interactions included stances such as "this is my patient and it is my right to discard any agreement reached in a meeting without consulting others" which have since evolved to stances reflecting a genuine sense of a need to consult with "the rest of the gang" before changing management plans.

Not all has been working smoothly. Paradoxically, the most stressful aspect of the project has been the challenge of protecting the professionals' ability to participate. The ACDU is an innovative project with (as yet) uncertain outcomes in an era of substantial economic challenges as well as staff shortages. The department managers involved have been reluctant to free resources to the ACDU, even though they are well aware of the necessity of quality improvement in the areas addressed by the project. The financing system does not encourage interorganizational dialogue and the development of shared responsibility for patients and diagnostic and treatment services. The two nurses in the ACDU both work half time for the project, but only one of the four participating doctors has time officially allocated to working in the ACDU. The others contribute on a voluntary basis – the ACDU exists in a pocket of good will, but currently lacks sufficient support for the long term. One important, but to the professionals of the team somewhat unfamiliar task, has been to initiate work strategically at securing resources for the ACDU's long-term survival and – possibly – expansion into a full-scale cancer diagnostic unit accepting referrals from all PHCCs in the Linköping University Hospital catchment area. Such a unit would be in line with the Commission's report, which states that comprehensive cancer services ought to be developed.

From a primary care perspective, the ACDU has provided a chance to discuss how PHCCs could best identify patients potentially suffering from gastrointestinal cancer in the population they serve. Members of the ACDU team are currently meeting with the PHCCs in order to learn more about their views on how the interface between primary and specialist care should be organized. These discussions have made evident the lack of systematic exchange of experiences among these professionals. The primary care professionals have also made clear that they believe that the ACDU could serve as a model for other areas where a close collaboration between various parts of the health-care system is necessary in order to provide the best care for each individual patient.

The ACDU has also highlighted several challenges inside the hospital-based specialist systems, such as the long waiting times for patients, especially for diagnostic services such as radiology and endoscopy. Also visible are problems related to the lack of communication with patients, which compromises the adaptation of care to individual patient needs (medical and others). Finally, as already noted, another system challenge is the financial support for interdepartmental and even interorganizational investigation units such as the ACDU.

The ACDU challenges the existing system in many ways, and it will be interesting to see how the system responds to these challenges. The project is slated to run for another 6 months. Hopefully, it will be seen as an intrapreneurial seed for organizational change, addressing all three corners of the triangle. (An intrapreneur is a person who focuses on innovation and creativity and who translates ideas into reality by operating within the organizational environment.) At the very least it should be seen as an example of what can happen when professionals wanting better work lives and organizational systems needing change are brought together in service of better outcomes for patients and populations.

Given the ultimate ambition with the ACDU and the entire regional collaboration – to improve colon cancer services across the spectrum of care – one question begs for an answer: Will the changes developed in the collaboration lead to better services and outcomes? The project seeks to address this challenge by way of performance measurement.

The Measurement Team

Informed by previous research suggesting that good measurement is essential for improvement efforts and their evaluation,[29,30] the demonstration project team set up a measurement team, with members drawn from the participating county councils. The idea here was to develop a balanced bouquet of measures that would indicate the state, and regional variation of colon cancer over time as well as signs of impact from improvement efforts initiated through the demonstration project. These "systems measures" are posted publicly, with regular updates, on the web. The group organized the measures according to the Clinical Value Compass model,[31] with some 20 measures in four domains, including the following examples.

1. Clinical outcomes:
   - the proportion of patients with colon cancer who have no reported post-operative complications, per county and quarter (*see* Figure 11.4)
   - relative 5-year survival, annual national data (based on mandatory reporting) stratified per county, for men and women.
2. Functioning; health status:
   - self-reported anxiety, appetite, quality of life; reported at the first visit after receiving the colon cancer diagnosis, and at the first post-operative visit.
3. Experience of services:
   - degree to which I have been able to participate in decision making about my care
   - degree to which I have received sufficient information about my condition.

4. Resources; costs:
    ● length of hospital stay for surgery
    ● costs for diagnostic assessment of patients with suspected colon cancer
      (whether confirmed or not).

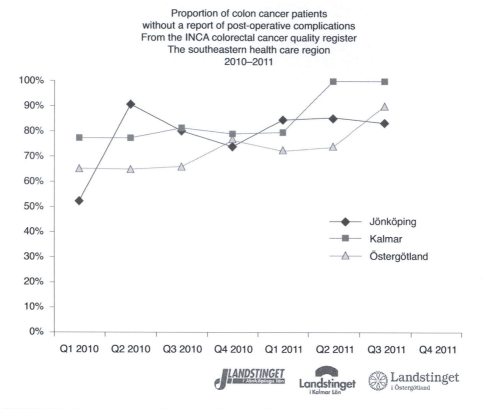

FIGURE 11.4 Quarterly proportions of patients without reported postoperative complications, by county council

Applicability of the Triangle Model in This Case and Beyond
••••••••••••

The efforts to improve colon cancer services in southeastern Sweden – from prevention, diagnosis, and therapy to palliative care – exemplify a number of ways that the triangle model applies also in this context. In fact, the model offers a unifying frame for connecting the many parallel changes underway in the region. A number of contextual circumstances enhance the model's applicability.

● The comprehensive nature of the health system: the fact that "population" is understood by actors throughout the system as *all* residents in the geographic area covered, and that "care" includes social as well as medical services, brings a different understanding of "everyone" to the table.

- The foundation for equity established by the existence of universal health care coverage, which enables anyone in need of care to access such care (even if, as highlighted in Swedish cancer services, too often with challenges of delay and fragmentation). Also of note is the willingness at the governance level to make promises about the care all residents can expect.

- The tradition of regional collaboration, particularly regarding tertiary care, the medical school, and the joint funding for clinical research throughout the region, helped nurture relationships across the region and among actors in its three distinct county council health care systems, providing a powerful basis for participation in this demonstration project.

- The extensive experience in many parts of the region of continuous improvement efforts, which paved the way for this innovative initiative to improve colon cancer services in a wide range of areas and ways. Examples include the adoption of a Breakthrough Series approach with joint learning seminars, peer learning, and action periods "at home"; the measurement team dedicated to develop the best possible indicators of colon cancer services performance over time; and the inclusion of patients and family members in the initiative.

- The active participation of volunteering patients and family members in regional learning seminars, who have shared their experience and interacted with clinicians and managers. In addition to adding a unique and central perspective on colon cancer care, they likely also remind participants of whom they are accountable to, not only in their daily clinical work, but also when they wrestle with improving their health care system. They provide faces and voices of the patient outcomes referenced in the model. This illustrates the ways in which "everyone" can become involved in the work of the triangle.

Professional development is integral to the triangle model. Arguably, most participants in the demonstration project are learning from their experience. Rather than issuing top-down directives for improvement, the regional leadership empowered local teams to experiment with ways to fulfill the promises made to residents and cancer patients in the region. Participants engage in developing new forms of collaboration, across boundaries of geography, specialty, and profession. They learn experientially about systematic improvement work, including the use of measurement over time, patient centeredness, and systems thinking. The joint learning seminars demonstrate the breadth of the challenges at hand, and the benefits of taking several complementary approaches to addressing them – for example, for early detection and timely diagnostic work-ups.

The work also adds new dimensions to participants' professional roles, as reported for instance by the participating professionals of the ACDU described earlier. The professionals involved state that one of the obvious strengths with the ACDU is that they have become "better cancer care workers" as they have benefitted from the discussions about cancer assessment and treatment with colleagues from other disciplines. For others in the demonstration project, participation is linked to an interprofessional master's program on quality improvement and leadership in health and social care run by The Jönköping Academy for Improvement of Health and Welfare (including faculty who are also co-authors of this chapter). They are actively involved in the project and contribute to it through practicums designed to apply theory to practice. Geared to mid-career professionals and managers, the master's program applies a blended learning design,[32] a mix of campus sessions and distance learning involving web-based study so that students can combine their studies with their regular jobs. The demonstration project includes two heads of radiology services in the region, a biomedical analyst and improvement advisor, a radiology nurse and a gastrointestinal surgeon, who are also students in the master's program.

Several participants in the demonstration project have, at different points, expressed confusion about the project design, about who is supposed to do what, and when. This may reflect the fact that it is not a small or trivial task to improve colon cancer services for a geographically defined population across a region with three distinct health systems. There is no established standard template to bring into the activity. It is noteworthy that (to the best of our knowledge) nowhere else in Sweden has any similar attempt to improve cancer care been set in motion. Based on our demonstration project observations, we suggest that the triangle model can serve as a unifying frame for large-scale improvement initiatives like this one. It can help remind participants – "everyone" – of the key *ends* – better health, better care, and better professional development – to work toward, while experimenting with different *means* for achieving them.

It may well be that to get at the work of real application of the triangle, you need to get a specific focus for improvement. Regional leaders and faculty from the three universities in the region had met regularly over several years to discuss cooperation, including multiple discussions about the triangle "in general" that didn't go anywhere. When they got "real" about a specific area – improvement of services for colon cancer – things began to happen: the proposal was developed collaboratively, and, when approved, the work got under way across the region. Timing is crucial. The reasons for why this unique demonstration project could happen *here* in Sweden *now* is that "everyone" went from talking to doing as they sunk their teeth into some real and pressing challenges. This hard work, which is by no means complete, is only possible when those involved are improving the systems where they work, learning and sharing meaningful information about real patient outcomes, and developing their professional knowledge and skills together.

Contributing A

On Working Together

The editors chose the theme: th
outcomes for individuals and pop
ity, safety, value; and better profe
mastery in their work. They and ot
from decades of personal involvem
ers, leaders, teachers, and researc

They invited the authors to jc
particular attention to an aspect, a
in the daily life of an academic m
and respected; some but not all of
to attend 90-minute monthly conf
A web-based platform supported
and emerging chapters, and facili
conferences started with the work
critical and formative commentary
ters, working from outlines or wr
and comment on the emergent w

This last chapter was written a
The editors conducted individual
authors about the way the theme
insights they had about the proce
tions was shared with the intervie
the later monthly conference calls

Acknowledgments

This chapter draws on the efforts of many participants in the demonstration project, including:

- leaders of the county level teams: Leni Lagerqvist, OT (Kalmar), Marie Lagerfelt, RN (Östergötland), and Urban Jürgensen, MD (Jönköping)
- Kjell Lindström, MD, PhD, at the primary care research and development unit in Jönköping and Peter Stålhammar, MD, a FP in Sävsjö, outside Jönköping
- improvement advisors, including Mari Bergeling Thorsell, Peter Kammerlind, and Ann-Margreth Kvarnefors (at Qulturum)
- Anna-Lena Nilsson, Carina Persson, and Eva Benzein (Kalmar) who undertook additional demonstration project research.

The research on the demonstration project is funded in part by the Swedish Association of Local Authorities and Regions (as part of the funding for the demonstration project) and by the Medical Research Council of Southeast Sweden.

References

1. Batalden PB, Davidoff F. What is "quality improvement" and how can it transform healthcare? *Qual Saf Health Care.* 2007; **16**(1): 2–3.
2. Government Offices of Sweden. *Health and Social Issues.* Stockholm: Government Offices of Sweden; 2008. www.sweden.gov.se/sb/d/3288/a/19569 (accessed August 11, 2011).
3. Swedish Ministry of Health and Social Affairs. *The Health and Medical Service Act (1982:763).* Stockholm: Ministry of Health and Social Affairs; 2003. www.sweden.gov.se/content/1/c6/02/31/25/a7ea8ee1.pdf (accessed August 11, 2011).
4. Government offices of Sweden. *Health and Medical Care in Sweden.* www.sweden.gov.se/sb/d/15660/a/183490 (accessed July 6, 2012).
5. Swedish Association of Local Authorities and Regions. *Open Comparisons.* Stockholm: Swedish Association of Local Authorities and Regions; 2010. http://english.skl.se/activities/open_comparisons (accessed December 15, 2011).
6. Swedish Association of Local Authorities and Regions, Swedish National Board of Health and Welfare. *Quality and Efficiency in Swedish Health Care: regional comparisons 2010.* Available at: www.skl.se/vi_arbetar_med/oppnajamforelser/halso-och_sjukvard_2/quality-efficiency-2010 (accessed August 11, 2011).
7. Wigzell K, Halle C, Hållén J, *et al. A National Cancer Strategy for the Future: Summary.* SOU 2009:11. Stockholm: Swedish Government Inquiries; 2009.
8. Statistics Sweden. *Sweden's Population Statistics for the First Half of 2011: Stockholm and Örebro.* 2011. www.scb.se/Pages/TableAndChart (accessed September 8, 2011).
9. http://mapfrappe.com/index.html
10. Andersson-Gare B, Neuhauser D. The health care quality journey of Jonkoping County Council, Sweden. *Qual Manag Health Care.* 2007; **16**(1): 2–9.
11. Ridderstolpe L, Johansson A, Skau T, *et al.* Clinical process analysis and activity-based costing at a heart center. *J Med Syst.* 2002; **26**(4): 309–22.
12. Sjodahl R, Lemon E, Nystrom PO, *et al.* Complications, surgical revision and quality of life with conventional and continent ileostomy. *Acta Chir Scand.* 1990; **156**(5): 403–7.

13. Strindhall M, Henriks G. How
    Sweden. *Qual Manag Health C*
14. Peterson A, Carlhed R, Lindal
    quality improvement and the u
    cardial infarction. *Qual Manag*
15. Flamm BL, Berwick DM, Kab
    a "breakthrough series" collabo
16. Kilo CM. A framework for c
    Healthcare Improvement's Bre
17. Leape LL, Kabcenell AI, Gan
    breakthough series collaborativ
18. Wenger E, McDermott RA, Sny
    ing knowledge. Boston, MA: H
19. Regional Cancer Center SHR. *i*
    löften.] Linköping: Regional Ca
    Verksamheter/Halso--och-vardu
20. Varadhan KK, Varadhan KK, L
    future of improving surgical car
21. Thomsen T, Villebro N, Møll
    Cochrane Database Syst Rev. 20
22. Griffin FA, Classen DC. Detec
    Tool approach. *Qual Saf Health*
23. Canslätt E, Sjödahl R. Adverse
    pilot study. *Presented at Utveckl*
24. Arriaga AF, Lancaster RT, Ber
    evidence-based best-practice a
    2009; **250**(4): 507–13.
25. American College of Gastroent
    of Gastroenterology; 2011. Avai
    (accessedDecember 16, 2011).
26. SBU – Swedish Council on H
    Cancer [In Swedish: Om scre
    at: www.sbu.se/sv/Publicerat/
    av-befolkningens-deltagande/l
    December 16, 2011).
27. Lindstrom K. Early detection of
    Tidig upptäckt av patienter m
    Seminar, Linkoping, Sweden, 2
28. Ekedahl S, Hauschildt P, Lind
    ate the early detection of pati
    Kan Stålhammars score under
    primärvården?] *Allmänmedicin.*
29. Ovretveit J, Staines A. Sustaine
    the Jonkoping quality program.
30. Thor, J. *Getting Going on Gettin
    healthcare organization? Implica*
    Stockholm: Karolinska Institute
31. Nelson EC, Mohr JJ, Batalden
    compass. *Jt Comm J Qual Impr*
32. Keller C, Stevenson K. Participa
    program in health care. *Int J We*

much more extensive involvement in the ongoing work of improving health care and new roles in developing professionals for the future. Further, the idea of "everyone" involved in settings where health care is publicly financed invites politicians and their representatives along with professionals and patients to the work of improving health care.

Closing Words

We came together aware of the themes of better outcomes, better system performance and better professional development and grew in our understanding of their interdependence. We grew in our understanding that to excel at any one of the "points" in the triangle, one must excel in them all. Systemic "linkage" of these three aims in health care means that underperformance in any one of them limits excellence in each of the others. As an integrated system taken together they can be transformative. Developing the "corners" of the triangle and their inextricable linkages as a system is the task for leaders in academic medical centers and in all health-care systems seeking the next level of excellence and systems of improvement that are both sustainable and generative.

Getting further clarity about these three aims, the linkages among them, and the invitation for all to participate in the work offers many opportunities. We offer this book in service of the continued vitality of those future efforts to improve health and health care. While this idea of an "integrated system of improvement" seems obvious in many ways to those of us involved in the construction of this book, we recognize that the full development and deployment of the idea will require the work of dedicated leaders, professionals, and patients to be more fully realized.

Index

Entries in **bold** denote references to figures or tables.

Index

Index